Grace Notes on Nursing

John Graham Pole

HARP The People's Press

H-ealing **A**-rt **R**-econciling **P**-eoples

Clydesdale, Nova Scotia, CANADA

HARP Publishing: The People's Press

216 Clydesdale Road,
Clydesdale, Nova Scotia,
Canada B2G 2K9

www.harppublishing.ca

harppeoplespress@gmail.com

Catalogue-in-Publication data is on file with the
Library and Archives Canada
ISBN: 978-1-990137-41-9

Cover Art: Barbara Farquharson Fry
Book Layout: Cathy Lin: wdesign68@gmail.com

The Circle of Abundance Indigenous Program, Coady International
Institute, St. Francis Xavier University: https://coady.stfx.ca/circle-
of-abundance; and David Suzuki Foundation (one nature): https://
davidsuzuki.org receive 20% of sales, distributed equally

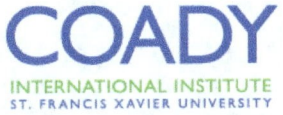
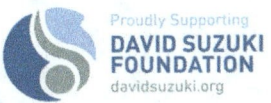
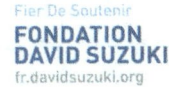

To my sister Mary, my first nurse teacher
And to every nurse I worked beside
in forty-plus years of doctoring:
My helpers, companions, teachers

Artist's Statement

Grace Notes on Nursing is a gift to my heart and the inspiration for this hooked rug. In attempting to capture the essence of the nurse-physician relationship, I reflected on my own extensive experience as a nurse.

This humble depiction speaks to the patient at the centre of care, the heart of caring, and the nurse-physician relationship. Hooked onto a background of healing green, and inspired by Florence Nightingale, is a stylized lamp symbolic of nursing. Its handle supports the physician's symbol of the Rod of Asclepius, the deity in Greek mythology associated with healing. The grace notes on the left refer to the book's title; the electrocardiogram speaks to the rhythm of the heartbeat of service in caring for those at the centre of care; and the image of the heart represents compassion for all.

Many thanks to the collaborative efforts of Jane Steele, owner of Riverhouse Rug Hooking Studio and Sue Cunningham, both rug hookers *extraordinaire*.

About the Artist

As a former staff nurse, educator, manager, author, and speaker for more than forty years I remain passionate about the art and the science of nursing and the quality of patient care. More recently, I discovered the powerfully reflective world of rug hooking. Art is created through quiet thoughts accompanying each hooked loop—and within this art there is healing.

Barbara Fry, BN, RN (ret'd), MAdEd

Praise for Grace Notes

Dr. Graham-Pole is a gifted storyteller. transporting us to a recounted moment that was salient for him. Each story is vivid and specific in detail, some more emotionally charged than others but all evoking a reaction, both visceral and cognitive. This book is brimming with wisdom and insights that guide, teach, inspire, and point the way to becoming the best one aspires to be. Dr. Graham-Pole has brought out of hiding this aspect of medicine's hidden curriculum by acknowledging the impact of nurses in shaping a doctor's identity and how they choose to practice their profession.

Laurie N. Gottlieb, RN, PhD, ScD(hon), FCAHS, FCAN
Professor, McGill University

Grace Notes is a love note to nursing. Delivered through the humble and inspired eyes of a physician as he reflects on his journey to embracing that showing up human and with a truly caring heart are treatments in and of themselves.

Sybil St. Claire
Professor of Theatre (Arts and Wellness), Goddard College,
Orlando, Florida

Here's something new: a doctor's experiences of working with nurses who became his teachers, mentors, colleagues, friends — and "ministering angels." Everyone of them was instrumental in the author's recognition of medicine as both art and science.

I much enjoyed reading *Grace Notes*. John is a fine writer with the power to draw the reader into each scene he describes, to let us see and feel what is happening. Each story comes alive through its vivid historical detail and its use of local dialect—be it West of Scotland or Southern US.

This is a memoir that is also an homage to the profession of nursing. These laudatory portraits include many touching moments as well as tense encounters with nurses who were unafraid to speak up and question a doctor's judgment.

John offers this prayer: "We can only hope there will be nurses like the ones portrayed in *Grace Notes* for us and our loved ones when our time of need comes."

Tilda Shalof, RN
Critical Care Nurse, Medical-Surgical ICU,
Toronto General Hospital for 36 years
Author of *A Nurse's Story—
Life, Death, and In-Between in an Intensive Care Unit.*

The world of nurse-physician relationships is a complex one frequently storied with dramatic themes of patients in clinical crises, gender and power dynamics, and romance. *Grace Notes on Nursing* is different. Written with notes of vulnerability, profound compassion, and deep respect, the book reveals a refreshing, lesser known, yet commonly practiced aspect of that professional relationship.

As a registered nurse for more than forty years serving in a variety of roles, I am profoundly grateful for the opportunity to gain insight into some of this marvelous physician-author's reflections on his learning journey. John Graham-Pole's eloquent homage to the grace notes of caring sung by nurses, is a must read. In other words, if you are looking for a deeper understanding into the inner world of healthcare relationships, this book may be just be what the doctor ordered!

Barbara Fry, RN (ret'd), BN, M. Ad. Ed

Grace Notes on Nursing is a wonderful tribute to the nurses who care for us from the day we are born to the day we die. It highlights the role of the nurse as a teacher, particularly to physicians. The lessons given are humanistic—that it is important and healthy to be close to your patients, that spending time getting to know them leads to better caregiver morale and more effective healing.

Dr. Graham-Pole emphasizes the healing role of humor, and describes a spontaneous marshmallow fight among nurses that beautifully encapsulates how having fun at critical moments can be the perfect salve for a bad week. *Grace Notes* underscores the strength and endurance of nurses who use their heads, hands and hearts to heal and experience with all their senses the lives of their patients when they are suffering the most and are at their most vulnerable.

An inspirational must-read for those pursuing careers in medicine.

William Slayton, MD, Professor and Chief
Division of Pediatric Hematology-Oncology,
Department of Pediatrics, University of Florida

Grace Notes on Nursing takes you on a journey through the experiences of retired pediatrics professor John Graham-Pole. He recounts stories of what he learned about caring from the nurses he has worked with. The nurses he witnessed in their caring work taught him that his purpose at the bedside was to attend, and to offer loving care to those in need.

John titles this touching tribute to the nursing profession *Grace Notes on Nursing* because nurses are both complementary and essential, just as are grace notes in a music composition. He asserts that nurses interweave the art and science of care more skillfully and easily than doctors, as they work equally with their heads, their hearts and their hands.

John weaves stories about influential nurses from the time he entered medicine as a resident doctor in 1963 at St. Bartholomew's Hospital in London, UK, to his retirement in 2007 at Shand's Children's Hospital at the University of Florida, where he was the pediatric director of the bone marrow transplant unit. He shares with his readers stories of the earliest nurses who impacted his future life as a doctor—his sister Mary, his aunts Ella, David and Joan, and "Auntie" Muriel and all those who nursed his family on their death beds. He shares personal stories of the nurses that he went on to learn from throughout his career—from the operating room nurse who taught him how to perform his first circumcision, to the midwives who guided him in delivering a baby, to the nurses who showed him how to care for the dying with dignity and compassion. He asserts that all the most important lessons in healthcare he learned from nurses.

These deeply personal and emotional stories will compel you to keep reading as we learn how John learned to move past his role as a doctor and diagnostician to a role more grounded in caring, and how he achieved this through the act of making vital time and space for his patients. As a nurse with nearly forty years of experience, I was deeply moved by John's descriptions of the caring traits he had witnessed. I have only once before in my career heard another doctor tell medical students to look for the nurse on the unit who seems to know the most and learn from them. Every chapter gives you another glimpse into Dr. Pole's journey to becoming a world-renowned physician and the nurses he credits for his success.

I recommend this book to anyone looking for a glimpse into the life of a physician and the stories that shaped him. It is a poignant acknowledgement of nurses' vital place in healthcare as caregivers and educators. In the current state of healthcare, and as nurses struggle to recover from the stressors of the pandemic, we need to feel valued and applauded for all we have endured. This book outlines all the reasons that nursing is so vital from the perspective of a physician who eloquently shares how integral they are. John repeats the following quote several times throughout the book—one I have often considered myself. So I will close with this tribute: *We're all potential patients: just hope there's a good nurse there for you when it happens.*

Carol Flegg, RN, M.Ad.Ed, PhD
Sessional Instructor in Nursing, University of Calgary and Brock University, St. Catharines

Grace Notes is a true testament to the millions of unsung heroes in the world. Those heroes cater to the needy, often at the worst times in their lives. Nurses are the backbone and spine of any healthcare system. They are friends, colleagues, teachers, learners, critics, challengers, collaborators, helpers, supporters and more all at the same time. Grace Notes makes you pause and think..... think and reflect about what it actually means to be a nurse! Far from being a cake walk, it takes a lion's heart, nerves of steel and tender hands full of compassion. It's a must-read for every medical professional! Dive in!

Ketan Kulkarni, MD,
Associate Professor of Pediatrics, Dalhousie University
Lead Author, Soar: A Soul's Quest

I loved this book! John is a storyteller who invites the reader into the room, into the moment and the feelings. There were passages when I laughed out loud, like the image of days gone by when John entered a ward to encounter the Head Sister with her two staff nurses perched on the edge of their seats, like ministering angels on either side of God. Then there were passages that made me weep because they evoked memories of patients and colleagues that I also carry.

John makes clear that it is nurses that taught him to stop and listen to what they could teach him. Nurses teach the value of the right balance between skill and empathy. Nurses hear the stories their patients crave to tell them. This in turn helps those patients make sense of their situation, which leads to their healing.

This book is authentic, humble, appreciative and true to the experiences of clinical care over many years. I have the urge to order cases of this book to give to every nurse I know!

Thank you, John, for writing *Grace Notes on Nursing*.

Barbara Heatley-O'Neill, RN, BScN, MAdEd
Certified Professional Co-Active Coach

In reading *Grace Notes on Nursing* one receives a gift of great wisdom from a master teacher. Dr Graham-Pole has dedicated his life to the loving care of others. He has done this at a time when physicians have been trained in a strictly biomedical model that has devalued the *art* of doctoring and the central role that *relationship* plays. In this volume, John reveals the central place that nurses have played in his development as a physician who has been on the front lines of pediatric oncology. The stories are intimate, humble, wise, humorous, poignant, entertaining, and full of love. Through sharing these memories John's teachers become our teachers, and the reader emerges with a renewed appreciation for the importance of loving care.

Mary Lynch MD FRCPC
Founder (Pain Medicine) Royal College Physicians and Surgeons, Canada
Professor of Anesthesia, Pain Management, Perioperative Medicine,
Psychiatry and Pharmacology,
Dalhousie University, Halifax, Nova Scotia

It is rare that one reads a physician's story written with such a profound understanding of professional nursing. John Graham-Pole has done just that. He honors and appreciates nursing in this deftly woven tale. Beautiful language and rich dialogue enliven the humanity of his characters. I was particularly drawn to his dialogue with Scottish folk when he was in medical training in the U.K. Humor and tenderness permeate his writing, creating a welcoming and heartwarming read.

There is great dignity in his storytelling as he speaks of his sister's early training as a nurse, and his own training by nurses, midwives, and nuns. Courage, confidence and humility permeate these pages as John addresses his care and treatment of children battling cancer. He does not shy away from his own vulnerability. A summary of the twenty-one lessons his nursing colleagues have taught him is present in these pages. It should be curriculum fodder for both doctors and nurses. A good read, this: you will cherish the blessings and rich moments of giving care.

Pamela Anna Teresa Micieli (Mitchell), M.F.A., R.N.
Writer and Nursing Consultant, Bend, Oregon

A lovely book, which really got me thinking. Hearing Dr. John Graham-Pole praise the profession of nursing reminds me to feel proud of the very real and human-centred work we do. At a time when nursing is more than ever moving into offices and away from the bedside, John shows us the really hard lifting of healthcare happens at the bedside. Those among us who have been patients know firsthand the art of nursing. For those who fortunately do not, they can read this lovely book to find out about it.

Kendra MacEachern RN, BScN, CHPCN(C)
Palliative Care/Oncology, St. Martha's Hospital, Antigonish, Nova Scotia

Nursing is an art form that requires a gentle balance and flow of communication and negotiation between the patients and their caregivers. The foundation of nursing is based on care, compassion and communication. In its holistic form it encompasses biopsychosocial needs, cultural preferences, and spiritual needs.

Dr. John Graham-Pole understands this deeply and embraces the knowledge of nurses. He is that gentle voice of engagement and trust. He is a champion of nurses and embraces the symbiotic relationships between patient, family, nurse, and physician.

In this, his latest book, *Grace Notes on Nursing*, John shares stories of how nurses have mentored and helped shape him into the physician he aspired to be. You will be inspired by his stories.

Maria van Vonderen RN., BSc.N. M.Ed.
Psychiatric Nurse, St. Martha's Hosptal, Antigonish, Nova Scotia

John Graham-Pole hits it out of the park with his book *Grace Notes on Nursing*. He completely masters the concept that nurses interweave the art, science and spirit of care. He unabashedly recognizes the shortcomings of most doctors who, when left alone, lack the connectedness and spirituality to lift patients up to a more meaningful plane. John paints a vivid picture for the reader of the critical difference between medicine and healing, and he tells the remarkable story of how nurses and not doctors shaped his spirituality and enhanced his connectedness to patients and families. This is a must read.

Michael S. Okun, M.D.
Adelaide Lackner Professor of Neurology
Executive Director, Norman Fixel Institute for Neurological Diseases
University of Florida Health

The old saw, "Nurses care, doctors heal," is quite inaccurate; both do both. I observed firsthand as this statement withered in the presence of Dr. John Graham-Pole, my friend. With his usual low key, professional and affable manner, John helped usher the old stereotype back into the dark arcane corners where it belonged.

I have viewed John from a distance, through the lens of a camera as he danced, sang, clowned, waxed poetic, and engaged in Olympic-level tomfoolery. He was genuinely present in every moment. My pictures captured moments of joy, sadness, elation and tender humanhood. All these times, John was not just playing a part, he *was* the part. He was the brilliant physician-scientist wearing the clown nose, he was the vulnerable doctor, he was the compassionate human being who embraced all the sorrow in the room and who did everything he could to soften some of life's harshest and cruelest blows. He is love, kindness, and a bit of a rascal. We ate and drank together frequently. We crashed and thrashed about on a racquetball court where I learned firsthand (and have the chipped tooth to prove it) that John has a very competitive athletic spirit. Who knew?

John is fluent in silence. Some of the best times we spent together were in silence, just being in each other's energy. A wry smile usually signaled the end of our "conversation." At the bedside with John, everybody knew that all opinions and skill sets were respected. He understood that in some moments, the most important thing was a cool, wet cloth and someone to hold the garbage can. John could and would gladly lend a hand with either task, all the while dictating orders for a medication dose to bring more relief. All of us nurses were colleagues, not subordinates.

In these stories, John points out time and again the role that his nursing colleagues, teachers, coaches, mentors, confidantes, caretakers and friends played in his growth as a physician and as a man.

He earned the respect of many in his circle by simply being humble and never losing sight of the fact that above all else, he is human. An extraordinary human being.

Steve Kavalin, CRNA
Anesthesiologists of Greater Orlando, Florida

Chapters

Foreword

When Dr. Graham-Pole approached me about a book he was writing praising his many nurse friends and colleagues for the countless lessons he learned from them over the course of his career as a doctor, I was intrigued. I was further intrigued by the title—*Grace Notes on Nursing*—a play on the title of Florence Nightingale's seminal work on nursing. What did the word "grace" mean in the context of Nightingale's title and why was it chosen? Once my curiosity was piqued, I agreed to look at Dr. Graham-Pole's book.

The book sat in my inbox for two weeks. Then, one Saturday morning, no longer able to procrastinate further, I began to read. I quickly became drawn into the stories and spent the most satisfying next few hours fully engrossed.

Dr. Graham-Pole is a gifted storyteller transporting us, the reader, in time and place to a recounted moment that was salient for him. Each story is vivid and specific in detail, some more emotionally charged than others but all evoking a reaction, both visceral and cognitive. These stories are about events—moments in time—ranging from ordinary, everyday encounters to life-defining experiences with nurses, colleagues, patients, and their families. Each had an impact, leaving an indelible mark on Dr. Graham-Pole in his 40-year quest to become a better, more caring, more compassionate, more self-aware physician and colleague.

This book goes beyond sharing interesting stories. As with all effective stories, it is brimming with wisdom and insights that guide, teach, inspire, and point the way to becoming the best one aspires to be.

Intentional and Attentional Choosing

Dr. Graham-Pole began his medical career in the 1960s. During these intervening years, the healthcare system has undergone considerable changes, owing to advances in scientific knowledge that underpin best practices, the advent of new technologies for diagnosis and treatment, advances in pharmacology and new treatment protocols, and the like. These changes have profoundly affected healthcare services and how both medicine and nursing are practiced. However, Dr. Graham-Pole reminds us that what have not changed are humans and their needs for: security and safety; belonging and connection; affirmation and affection; being understood, accepted, and treated with dignity and compassion. These needs are ever more acutely felt during periods of vulnerability, uncertainty, fear, dependency, loneliness, emotional rawness, and threat—the familiar companions of illness, disability, injury, trauma, aging. How these needs are addressed depends on how nurses and doctors ***choose*** to show up in their respective roles; for it is a choice—what they *choose* to pay attention to—how they *choose* to be present and engage in a given situation—how they *choose* to connect with colleagues and another person, often a stranger who is in need of their knowledge and skills.

This book pays homage to nurses and their nursing. It lays bare why nurses are the most trusted profession by the public, as consistently reported in yearly Gallup polls. Observing, learning from, witnessing, being instructed by nurses, were all formative in how Dr. Graham-Pole *chose* to practice medicine. He *chose* to pay attention to nurses—an intentional choice—proving himself to be an astute, attentive, and reflective learner. He not only listened to what nurses were telling him but observed what they did, how they did it, and the impact they had on their patients.

Seeing Not Just Looking

As the philosopher Henry David Thoreau observed: *It is not what you look at that matters but what you see.* To see requires humility, an openness to learning, a curiosity to delve deeper, a sensitivity to the ecosystem in which one works, and an ability to reflect on what one has witnessed, experienced, and heard.

Dr. Graham-Pole *saw* nurses and nursing and peeled back the layers of what, on the surface, has been invisible to many, judged to be less complex than medicine, thus requiring less knowledge and skills. He *saw* just the opposite. He recognized the complexity involved in almost every nursing act, the creativity required to respond to challenges and find solutions. He was able to distinguish nursing as distinct from medicine rather than its extension. He witnessed nurses in their multitude of roles—supporter, nurturer, comforter, protector, advocator, educator, manager, supervisor. To name but a few.

He was able to *see* that at the heart of nursing was its relationship with patients. Nurses have been effective because they made the nurse-patient relationship central to their practice. It has been too easy to ignore, negate, or devalue the impact of kindness, compassion, caring, empathy, engagement when compared to what doctors do. That is, up until now. There is a growing body of scientific research that has provided much needed evidence that compassionate relational care makes a difference to patients' recovery AND is also economically beneficial in measurable ways (e.g., Trzaciak & Mazzarelli, 2019).

Dr. Graham-Pole *saw* the depth and breadth of nursing knowledge and interpersonal and technical skills. In 1978, Barbara Carper, in her now classic publication, identified the four fundamental patterns of *knowing* in nursing: empirical (science-based), personal (self-awareness), ethical (ethical, moral comportment), and aesthetic (transformative acts, art, imagination) (Carper, 1978; www.nursology.org). Christina Tanner, a nurse scholar known for her model of clinical reasoning, wrote about yet another type of knowing—the importance of knowing the patient. As Tanner explained "central to knowing is knowing the patient—their typical pattern of responses and knowing the patient as a person. Knowing the patient is central to skilled clinical judgment, requires involvement, and sets up the possibility for patient advocacy and for learning about patient populations" (Tanner et al., 1993).

Nursing has suffered by having lived for so long in medicine's shadows. Dr. Graham-Pole has made visible what nurses do and how they do it. He has held up a mirror for everyone to see the beauty in nursing, the creativity and complexity involved.

Acknowledgement and Gratitude

And this brings me to a major thread woven throughout—nurses as educators, the unsung and unrecognized heroes of medical education.

Since hospitals became the centre of the healthcare system, with nurses assuming the major role for keeping the system operating 24/7, nurses have been junior doctors' mentors, supervisors, and teachers. They have showed junior doctors the ropes—directing them to what to pay attention to, pointing out to them the early warning signs of deterioration, correcting their misinterpretations of signs and symptoms, suggesting diagnoses and the like. They have not only protected young doctors from committing avoidable errors, but have done all this to protect and safeguard their patients. Yet nurses have never been formally recognized nor given credit for their role in a doctor's medical training.

In recent years, much has been written about the hidden curriculum, that is, the curriculum that educators and mentors teach students without even realizing it through their interactions, modeling in the classroom and practice settings. The hidden curriculum consists of those unspoken values, beliefs, assumptions, norms—ways of being and ways of doing—espoused in the classroom that are either enacted or not, supported or contradicted. Dr. Graham-Pole has brought out of hiding this aspect of medicine's hidden curriculum by acknowledging the impact of nurses in shaping a doctor's identity and how they choose to practice their profession.

Who might benefit from Dr. Graham-Pole's experiences, insights, and wisdom?

Nurses: This gift of appreciation underscores why, what, and how nurses make a difference that often have profound long-lasting effects. Nurses can take great pride in their chosen profession.

Doctors: This book is a call to doctors to pay attention to what nurses do as there is much to be learned from them on how to be better doctors.

Students of medicine, nursing and healthcare professionals: This book is a call to be curious about what other fellow healthcare students are being taught. It is during these formative years that the foundations for future meaningful collaboration, authentic partnership, and effective teamwork are set, anchored in respect for the other's unique role and contributions to the healthcare enterprise.

The public: The stories in this book will trigger memories for all those who have had contact with nurses, both positive and negative. This book is a call to action to advocate for the types of nursing they had, or wished they had.

In Conclusion: A Note on the Word "Grace"

I began this foreword intrigued with why the word *Grace* was chosen to be part of the title of the book. Dr. Graham-Pole addresses my question in the first and last pages of his book. As he explains in the introduction, "*Grace Notes* are brief musical notations that precede the sounding of the longer note called the *principal.* A grace note may be complementary to that principal note—but it is harmonically and melodically essential." He ends his book, returning to the word *Grace:* "That beautiful word *Grace* derives from the Latin *gratia*, and means bestowing a service, or a gracious act that merits thankfulness. … The closely related word *gracious* implies one who offers courtesy, compassion, generosity of spirit, and mercy. "

Dr. Graham-Pole has himself been gracious and generous in this, his ode to nurses and their nursing, providing the important "grace" note to the art that Florence Nightingale recognized in nursing and its practice that embodies "grace."

-Laurie N. Gottlieb, RN,PhD, ScD(hon), FCAHS, FCAN
Professor, McGill University, Ingram School of Nursing,
Montreal, 2023

References
Carper, B. (1978). Fundamental Patterns of Knowing in Nursing".
Advances in Nursing Science. **1** (1): 13–24. doi:10.1097/00012272-197810000-00004. PMID 110216. S2CID 36893665.
Tanner, C.A., Benner, P. & Chesla, C. (1993). The phenomenology of knowing the patient. Image: *Journal of Nursing Scholarshi*p, 25(4), 273-280.
Trzaciak, S. & Mazzarelli, A. (2019). Compassionomics: *The revolutionary scientific evidence that caring makes a difference.* Pensacola, Fl: Studer Group.

CHAPTER 1

A Note on my Title

Nursing is an art ... as hard as any painter's or sculptor's work
- Florence Nightingale

Dirty, gritty, messy, grinding, brutal, rough, heartbreaking—also inspiring, exhilarating, fun

- Tilda Shalof

Grace Notes are brief musical notations that precede the sounding of a longer more prominent note called the *principal*. A grace note may indeed be complementary to that principal note—but it is harmonically and melodically vital. This describes for me the working relationship between doctors and nurses. I felt it on every hospital ward round I ever made—first as a wet-behind-the-ears medical student in January 1963 on the hallowed wards of St. Bartholomew's Hospital, London, and last as I made my last goodbye rounds in June 2007 as a hoary attending doc on the Shands Hospital children's wards in Gainesville, Florida. St. Bartholomew's (Bart's) celebrated its eight-hundredth anniversary this year with a service of remembrance, sorrow, and gratitude at St. Paul's Cathedral; Shands is just sixty-five years old.

My title is a riff, too, on Florence Nightingale's *Notes on Nursing*, which she wrote in 1859 and which became the bible for the profession for which she was the trailblazer. The Lady of the Lamp called nursing an art "as exclusive a devotion, and as hard a preparation, as any painter's or sculptor's work." Two days after her death in 1910 the Lord Mayor of London christened Florence Nightingale "the greatest Englishwoman who ever lived." I think of the profession she championed as first and foremost an *art*, though it is incontestably a *science* too. And once I learned to stop and listen to what those nurses had to teach me, I knew we doctors must also become *artists* in attentive care at least as much as *scientists* who seek new cures.

But oh dear, did I get the wrong message—right from the start, in my very first medical school class. My primary task, my earliest doctor-mentors taught me, was *to diagnose and treat for cure* every patient who came under my hands. And that those hands I laid upon them were strictly for that very diagnosis which could alone lead to successful curative treatment. I was halfway through my career before I acknowledged just how far short of the truth this dictum fell: that the crucial purpose of my presence at the bedside must be as an attentive witness, offering loving care to every patient who came to me in need.

Nurses interweave this art, science, and spirit of care more effortlessly and very often more skillfully in their work than do we doctors. No amount of scientific knowledge and training could nor should ever replace this fundamental truth.

It was nurses—my colleagues, my friends, and my mentors—who taught me this life lesson.

CHAPTER 2

"A Good Case for the Perfesser"

There were two nurses—one senior and one very junior—who became those first mentors during my very earliest apprentice-ship in the science and art of medicine. The first happened along when I was a wet-behind-the-ears first-year med student. My second came four years on in 1967, at the start of my internship on the women's oncology ward.

I have a stark memory of peeking my head cautiously around the door of Annie Zunz Ward in 1963, knowing better than to enter without the ward sister's explicit permission. Sister Annie Zunz was sitting bolt upright behind an ancient mahog-any desk that faced directly away from the door. Starched white apron stretched tightly over dark Newcastle Blue ankle-length dress. To left and right, staff nurses on the edge of their seats: ministering angels on either side of God.

I cleared my throat and asked permission to enter. The conversation promptly broke off and the white veil-cap in-clined forward brief inches, which I took for assent. The ward stretched before me, two lines of beds as spick-and-span and precisely spaced as an army barracks awaiting the brigadier-gen-eral's inspection. The patients lay recumbent, immobile, loath to disturb the apple-pie order. I counted mutely as I ventured forward, clutching Mrs. Lovell's voluminous charts.

As I introduced myself to my newly assigned patient, I glanced at the nurse whom Sister Annie Zunz had seen fit to assign as my chaperone. As she stood mute and still on the other side of the bed I, struck mute in my turn, took in her ravishing beauty. Thick copper-colored hair pulled back tightly under grey probationer cap rested like a halo upon the face of an angel.

Her devastating prettiness, in such utter contrast to that of my patient, eighty-six-year-old Mrs. Lovell, stirred me to my core. I strived furtively to read off the name on her badge, bringing my gaze into direct line of sight of her left breast. I instantly averted my eyes, felt the heat rise up my face. Finally she moved to fold down Mrs. Lovell's sheets and I swiveled my mind abruptly back to the job in hand. She eased down the straps of our patient's flannel nightgown, which dropped promptly to the waist, baring the droop of ancient breasts. As my enchantress eased Mrs. Lovell down to a supine posture, the weighty protrusion of her abdomen leapt out at me, contrasting dramatically with the reed-thin arc of her ribs.

Surely she doesn't qualify for obesity… and I can safely rule out pregnancy… so all I need now is to recall the other twenty-plus causes of a protuberant abdomen.

I laid a tentative hand over where her liver should be, started to slide it downwards. I had almost reached her groin before my pinkie abutted against a firm edge; it had to be the bottom of her liver. Mrs. Lovell broke her silence.

"Feel it, dearie, do you? Big bugger, in'it?"

"Yes, er, yes, it is… er, big."

As I continued to grope I took in a cluster of puncture marks on Mrs. Lovell's skin below and to the left of her liver. Having broken her silence, Mrs. L. now became a treasure trove of priceless prompts.

"I spec' they'll be 'aving you stick a needle or two in me if you're goin' to be me new doctor."

"You've had other students put needles in your tummy, then, Mrs. Lovell?"

"Oh, dearie, yus, plen'y."

"You wouldn't have any idea why, would you, by any possible chance?"

"Well, bless me, yus! Thought you'd never ask, love. Like I said, it's me liver. It may be a big 'un but it ain't workin' worth tuppence nowadays. Ever since me 'epatitis."

The penny jangled to the floor. I took a closer look at her skin. Yellow as custard! How *could* I have missed it? Not what you'd call golden, but... no doubt about it, *she's lemon all over*. Striving to curb my glee, I turned to scrutinize her eyelids, lowering each one for a closer look. The white parts weren't white at all but just as lemony as the rest of her. I grew giddy at the thought of how close I had come to missing the signs that Mrs. Lovell's liver was failing fast.

"You'll be tellin' the perfesser all about me case in the mornin', then? 'E'll be sure to want to 'ear about me bleedin'."

"Bleeding?"

"Oh yus, that's why they rushed me in 'ere this time. I was bringin' up all this blood, and I got to feelin' giddy all over, I did. Me old man 'ad to ring up for a *nambulance*! They 'ad to empty me stummich out, an' gimme me this blood transfusion. They think it's stopped nah. The bleedin', that is."

I glanced back up at the nurse. In my elation, I had by some miracle let her slip briefly from my awareness.

"Er, nurse, I don't think I'll need you as my chaperone any more. I'm just going to have a nice long chat with Mrs. Lovell, see what else she thinks I should know about her... her case."

Now Mrs. Lovell was pulling on the sleeve of my pristine white coat, pointing with her other hand at a scattering of marks on her arms and hands. Pinkish circles, four or five each side, a spidery lacework extending outwards; they were like tiny spring flowers.

"They're allus peerin' an' pokin' at these 'ere thingummies on me skin an' all, doc. Dunno 'ow long they been there."

Oh, God, what on earth are those called? Spider something... An inescapable sign of liver trouble.

I could hardly wait to get at my *Cecil and Loeb Textbook of Medicine* before morning rounds and become the world's expert on liver failure. As I scooted back into the corridor heading for the library, I almost ran full tilt into my nurse chaperone. She was supporting a tenuous tower of bed pans, which did nothing to diminish her ravishing beauty. I made a clumsy attempt to hold the door open. She paused. My hopes rose. Then plummeted. Her words came out not as the looked-for murmur of thanks but as the outraged snarl of a lioness.

"Mrs. Lovell may be a *good case* for the professor's rounds tomorrow. But you might not have shown such *conspicuous* delight at spotting what's wrong with the poor woman. She might well not make it in here next time she bleeds."

I stood chastened to immobility as she swept past me into the ward. *A good case:* the words continued to echo in my mind throughout the morning. She had nailed me. If I faced right up to it, I really didn't care that much if Mrs. Lovell died on my watch. Just as long as she made it to Professor Scowen's rounds in the morning. And I had been far more consumed with this sexy young nurse than with the ancient woman in the bed. Just what kind of doctor was I going to be?

That day I made my commitment: I would stop and listen to every nurse who worked with me, regardless of whether it was their responsibility to teach me. That probationer had seen it as her job to take me down a peg, to force me to reflect on the truth of the situation. That we were both there at Mrs. Lovell's bedside as *caregivers*—and our roles were not that different. She was *our* patient, looking to *us* in need. Nothing wrong with my healthy lust for a gorgeous young woman, but there was a time and place for it—and this was decidedly not now. Now was the time to bring my caring attention to bear on my patient.

Thank you, forever unnamed nurse, for grasping that moment, your arms weighted with a wardful of bedpans, to teach me compassion.

CHAPTER 3

Opiates

The second enduring lesson my nurse colleagues had in store for me came soon after I started my internship on the men's oncology ward, working for Gordon Hamilton Fairley, Britain's first professor of medical oncology. Everything about my apprenticeship with the great man was daunting, but one of the senior staff nurses seemed to be watching out for me. She waylaid me early one morning in the sluice.

"Have you thought of writing Jeffrey for opiates? He's got to get some relief soon—the radiation's not helping him one jot."

The eighteen-year-old's cancer had spread from his femur to both hips, and on up to invade his lumbosacral spine. I could hardly bring myself to look at the devastation it had wrought that was so horrifyingly apparent on his Xrays. I had had to bite my lips to hold back tears when I first admitted him. I felt those tears once more welling in my throat at this nurse's kindness.

"Well, I wasn't sure I *could.* I mean, it might make it harder for them to tell if the radiation was working. Anyway, isn't morphine just for terminal cases?"

"It'll be just fine, John. The radiotherapists leave all these kinds of things to you interns."

"But won't he get hooked on the stuff?"

Staff held me in her steady gaze. She had caring eyes. And it was the first time anyone had used my Christian name since I'd started internship. It took me a long moment to realize the absurdity of my words. The tears were threatening to betray me.

"How long do you think he's going to be around?" she said finally. "That radiation is strictly for pain relief—and it hasn't done a damn thing for him so far."

"Thanks," I muttered. "I've been really worried about him."

I checked the precise dose of morphine. *What if I found him dead from an overdose in his bed tomorrow morning?* I was embarrassed to quiz her any more, though I sensed she'd have been tactful towards my oh-so-fragile ego. I ended up writing up Jeffrey for the smallest dose, but at Staff's urging I made it *t.i.d.*—three times a day—continuously.

"So he won't have to ask for it each time. And regular dosing works much better."

Yet another thing no one had told me in my Pharmacology & Therapeutics classes.

I hurried to check on Jeffrey as soon as I arrived on the ward next morning. He was sitting up in bed looking unusually perky. He greeted me before I could speak—with a grin. Something I'd never expected to earn from this angry hurting hulk of a man.

"Doc, that new medicine, the sweet-tastin' one. It's really 'elpin'. I got to sleep last night easy."

"Well, that's just great to hear, Jeffrey. Not feeling too sleepy, are you? No trouble breathing?"

"Nah. Even 'et me breakfast. And I made it onto the bedpan wivvat any 'elp!"

Ten day later, the senior resident from Radiotherapy caught up with me.

"Our patient is ready for discharge. He seems to be doing a whole lot better."

Not just your rads, buddy. That wouldn't explain his newfound cheeriness—or his hearty appetite.

Staff leant close to my ear: "Make sure you write him for five-hundred mills of morphine to take home. That'll last him even if they don't renew his prescription."

I went over my newly learned instructions with Jeffrey. "Make sure you've got the exact dose now. Three times a day regularly—but no more. And bring this bottle to Outpatients so they can refill it. Um… I don't think they know you've been taking it all this time."

"Thanks, doc." Another grin. "I feel real chipper."

I'd thought I was going to kill him with that stuff. Where would I have been without Staff's guidance? As I sat to write up Jeffrey's discharge notes, I offered up a prayer of thanks to Florence Nightingale's granddaughters. It was the nurses who actually made people better. Every one of us is a potential patient. I just hope there's a good nurse around when it happens to me.

CHAPTER 4

1950: A Nurse's Story

I come from a long line of nurses. It came as a surprise one December afternoon to realize I could use all the fingers on my left hand to count them: my elder sister Mary, my aunts Ella, David, and Joan—these are just the ones I know about. Then there were those who nursed my family members on their death beds: Auntie Muriel, my best friend Mike Trapnell's aunt, who cared for my mum; and the nurses in Cardiff and Newcastle-on-Tyne whom I got to thank in brief teary unions soon after my Aunt Ella and my dad had died. If nurses declared their professional credentials on *ancestry.com*, as doctors like to, I'll bet I'd find a whole lot more in my family tree. Which begs the question: *Why then did I become a doctor?* Ah! That's another story for another book...

My sister Mary was my first nurse teacher. When she was five years old our dad asked her: "What are you going to be when you grow up?" Mary answered without hesitation: "I'm going to be a nurse and I'm going to Bart's." This would have been in 1941 and Bart's was where our dad went to medical school. Sure enough, thirteen years later Mary entered Bart's Nurse Training School in Hertfordshire. When she told me this story, she added that of course she'd have known nothing of nursing at such a tender age. It had to have been a subconscious decision—just as was my own as a twelve-year-old to become a doctor and wipe out cancer after our mother died from that horrific disease. [Read more on this in my first memoir, *Journeys with a Thousand Heroes*].

Mary did indeed start to hone her ambition as a five-year-old, because a girl named Grace was evacuated from the slums of south-east London to our Devonshire home where

Dad had set up his rural practice. The evacuation of children in World War II—known as *Operation Pied Piper*—was designed to protect them from the risks of aerial bombing of the big cities. Mary remembered seven-year-old Grace in those days as "thin—white—pinched—dirty—poor—and very unhappy." She was covered in fleas, which our father swiftly dispatched with a mix of baking soda and lemon juice.

Fledgling nurse Mary had to teach Grace what a toothbrush was, and how to use it; up until then the only thing that little Eastender had ever known was a rag dipped in salt and rubbed once a week across her gums. At first the two of them had a hard time understanding each other, because this was well before Mum sent Mary off for Elocution lessons with Miss Sybil Athelstane Cox. So my big sister's Devonshire brogue and Grace's Cockney-sparrow dialects would have been foreign tongues to each other.

Before she died in 2022, just before her eighty-sixth birthday due on Christmas Day, Mary wrote her own "Notes on Nursing." Her very first bedpan encounter was during a preliminary nursing course she took at Weston General Hospital when she was sweet seventeen. The hospital stood outside the town to which we had moved after our parents divorced, when I was two and Mary was seven. She would have taken the longish daily bus ride to the hospital to report for bedmaking and bedpan cleaning duties. They presented her with a certificate at the end of the course, which stood her in good stead because it exempted her from the preliminary exams when she got accepted to Bart's Nursing School.

I picture Mary cutting open the big cardboard box that would have arrived from the shop where the nurses' uniforms were made according to the measurements Mummy had supplied: the traditional blue pinstripe uniform, hem stretching at least to mid-calf, together with cap, cape, aprons, bibs and all the other essentials for a nurse about to enter "The Royal and Ancient," as Bart's was always known. How did those nurse uniforms evolve? They speak to nurses being *service* workers much more than *knowledge* workers—that they exercised their hands more than their heads. The truth of course is that nurses have always worked equally with their heads, their hands, and their hearts.

My sister Mary's first day of nurses' training fell on August 29, 1955. She was assigned to a pokey little bedroom with another eighteen-year-old. As she carefully hung her starched probationer uniform, she would have arranged a few treasured possessions from home to keep her memories alive of her Somerset childhood. No Mum to accompany her, while the other forty-two nurse hopefuls all had family lingering long after the two Sisters who ruled the roost had started to shoo them out. Mary never told any of her new friends that she was essentially an orphan, our mother having died six months earlier when she was seventeen and I was twelve. But after a bit they noticed the absence of weekly letters and food parcels from home, and Heather, Josie and Sue started inviting Mary to spend their days off with them.

Mary quickly got into the swing of her new life, though she may have struggled with all the coursework. Science was not her strong point, any more than it was mine. Did she cram through the night like me, after copying by rote off the blackboard every chemical formula, every physics equation? For Sister Shorthouse was fond of telling her expectant class, "You may have chosen Bart's, but Bart's has not yet chosen you!"

But that first hurdle of basic sciences behind her, Mary graduated to the nearby annex left over from World War Two for her first taste of ward duty. First, the chest ward with Sister "Biggy" Biggs—TB, lung cancer and—primitive by today's standards—heart surgery. Mary's first encounter with death was that of a twelve-year-old boy after yet another attempt to repair his congenital heart malformation; the child's forty-plus-year-old parents sat through the night with him until he died at 3.45 am, as the blackbirds announced the dawn and the cockroaches awoke for their day in the ward kitchen.

Mary's move from the annex in St. Albans to the hospital proper was a blur of different specialties, but the patients were always the same in their respect and gratitude for the attention of their pretty young nurse. On the "abdominal ward," where cheery Cockney men nursed their hernias, she learned to relieve their sluggish bowels, as often as not manually. They never failed to reward her with boxes of chocolates when it came time for their discharge home. This was long before the discovery of *Helicobacter Pylori,* now known as the commonest cause of peptic ulcers and mostly treated successfully with antibiotics. In the nineteen-fifties Bart's head surgeon, Mr Birnstingle, made his reputation by curing gastric ulcers through total gastrectomy— an extremely radical operation that is rarely called for today.

On the neurosurgical ward Mary nursed a young Italian, Remo, who had suffered horrific injuries in a motorbike accident and remained in coma for many weeks. One morning, Mary was at the end of her night shift when she noticed Remo's eyes following her movements around his bed; he went on to make a spectacular recovery. But there was nought to be done for Mr. Ferriby, a consultant surgeon from "a lesser London hospital" (Bart's was one of the snobbiest of London's ten teaching hospitals). He had a cancer in his colon that had become too extensive to resect. It was rumoured that none of the house staff had ever plucked up the courage to perform a rectal examination on this senior member of the medical profession.

Mary remembered Mr. Ferriby with great affection because she qualified from probationer to official nurse status while she was "specialing" him, and she had just bought herself an EPNS buckle for her new navy blue Petersham belt. The £28 was all she could afford to pay, but Mr. Ferriby told her it wasn't good enough for such a caring and skillful nurse. After he was discharged home, surely to die very soon, a parcel arrived for Mary: he had bought her a superb buckle of pure silver decorated with cherubs. She kept both buckles until she herself died nearly seventy years later. I feel a glow of pride today that my big sister was feted for her newfound skills by one of my own profession.

Visiting hours in the 1950's were limited to two hours a day—an hour in the afternoon and one more in the early evening. The hordes of impatient family members surged through the ancient Henry VIII gateway to sit stiffly at bedsides, every patient's bed immaculate, both patients and family loathe to perturb the pristine order. It gave Mary a well-earned chance to join her nurse friends in the sluice, where they would arrange the higgledy-piggledy bunches of flowers that relatives brought from nearby Covent Garden flower market. Sometimes the nurses themselves would pass through the market on their way to work and bring a garland of flowers to one of their patients whom she had noticed never had any visitors.

But even when she became a fully licensed nurse Mary still had to show respect to anyone of senior rank—a nursing sister or most especially a consultant physician—by coming promptly to a halt, pressing herself against a nearby wall, and doffing her cap until they had passed by. Once a week early on Thursday mornings every nurse who could be spared scurried through the wards cleaning out grubby patient lockers, unwrinkling every sheet to pristine newness, and laying immaculately tidied case notes on each bed table. Anything resembling a lump or crumple in the bed linen might perhaps damage the fragile skin of a bedbound patient. This ritual had to be completed in time for the hospital's senior consultant physician, Sir Ronald Bodley Scott, to appear for rounds of the hospital on the dot of ten.

Sir Ronald would be accompanied by Matron, several senior Sisters, junior consultants and registrars, while the team of house staff, junior nurses and medical students brought up his train. This was back when Dr. Jim Malpas—who succeeded Sir Ronald as head of oncology and twenty-one years later hired me as a new consultant—was the great man's intern. It was Jim's duty to stand in the square waiting for the Rolls Royce to pull into its dedicated parking spot. Jim would then swing open the door for Barts' most distinguished physician and accompany him to the wards. The only exception to this strict punctuality came when Sister Dalziel received an early morning phone call from Sir Ronald announcing that he would be "running a trifle late." On these occasions he would invariably arrive dressed in a morning suit, complete with tails and pinstripe trousers. Everyone knew exactly what this signified: he had driven directly from Buckingham Palace where he served as physician to the household of King George VI, and subsequently that of Queen Elizabeth II.

Mary had a particular friend from her nursing student class, Josie Vincer, of whom she had loving memories: "A pretty elfin face, freckles, green eyes, and above all a vivacity and zest for life, with whom I shared a love of the countryside, flowers and beauty." At the age of twenty-seven Josie was struck down with multiple sclerosis, and the crippling disease dominated her life for the next forty years. Despite it she married Peter, a carpenter whom she met while working in her wheelchair in the Bart's Sick Rooms. She birthed a daughter, Petrina, who cared for Josie for the rest of her life. Mary remained Josie's devoted friend and gave a moving eulogy at her funeral: "The memory of her courage and endurance against such adversity will live with me forever."

It's impossible for me to imagine sharing such a friendship with another medical student from my 1966 graduating class. Is it just the difference between men and women—learned or inherent? My closest professional friendships have always been with nurses. Some of them as boyfriend and girlfriend, once as husband and wife, but mostly through close kinship between colleagues willing to push through the barriers that our two professions impose on themselves. In fifty years of training and practice, the balance that my nursing friends and I struck between deep professional commitment and wildly hilarious fun are among my most enduring.

CHAPTER 5

My Aunts

Auntie David was my father's youngest sister, and a member of Queen Alexandra's Royal Army Nursing Corps, established soon after World War II. I met her only half a dozen times, but I loved her matter-of-fact no-nonsense friendliness. I have a photo of her standing to attention in her army nursing uniform. I salute her right back: I may be a longtime pacifist but some of my best friends have been soldiers.

What did I learn from Auntie David? That you didn't have to be a sweet dimpling angel to be a highly skillful nurse. There was a maleness about her demeanor—ironic that she was always known by her second name (she was christened Muriel David). I wish I'd taken advantage of all the mentorship she could have given me; but back then the idea of nurses teaching doctors—actual or to-be—just hadn't entered my head, or my heart. Well, when the pupil is ready the teacher appears—and I wasn't ready. Perhaps we'll meet again in celestial conversation. Nice idea, eh?

It was only with Florence Nightingale that *women* began entering the nursing profession in any numbers. In ancient Rome and Alexandria nurses were mostly men, and still today in Africa men make up the majority of the profession. And it was men who were the nurses—albeit makeshift and with no professional training— in 1981 on Ward 5B of San Francisco Hospital when the first deaths from AIDs were being seen. Though yet to be identified or reported with any authority. The professional nurses were either forbidden or too scared to enter the ward where the horrors of this mysterious infection were a daily occurrence. It was those men who themselves became the make-do nurses:

they were the only ones available to wash and feed their dying brothers and lovers, and dress their horrific sores. Until they in their turn came to be nursed by their still healthier brothers upon their deathbeds. It feels like the deepest irony in the archives of disease that such beautiful young human beings should become so uglified in such numbers.

When I was twelve years old, the year my mother died, I went to Epsom College, a boys-only independent boarding school near London. It was then that I got to know my Aunt Ella. Aunt Ella was Mummy's first cousin, Aunt Jessie's daughter. Aunt Jessie lived her whole life in or near Newport in South Wales, but Aunt Ella left home early to study nursing in England, and somewhere in her youth cultivated a posh English upper-class voice. She lived outside London and commuted every day to Oxford Circus, where she was the senior nurse in charge of a huge TB clinic.

In the nineteen-fifties, tuberculosis was still rampant, especially in the overcrowded and unsanitary parts of southeast London. A born extrovert, Aunt Ella had no trouble raising her voice to speak to a whole room of people at once, not just at work but more especially in pubs and wine bars, where she honed her taste for gin and tonics and English Bitter.

The first time I met her was through a letter she sent me soon after I started at Epsom and a year after Mummy's ashes had settled in their urn. Aunt Ella and her husband Uncle Roger wanted to come to our annual Founder's Day, which took place near the end of the summer term. I had just had my thirteenth birthday, and I sat with Uncle Roger in companionable silence as we watched together Epsom College's first XI cricket team play their rivals from Eastbourne College. The only intrusion upon our silence, beyond the twitter of starlings in the surrounding beeches and the wonderful monotony of willow bat striking durable leather ball, was the sporadic sound of Aunt Ella regaling bemused schoolmasters amid their high pitched gales of laughter. She was the funniest woman I'd ever met—or hoped to meet—until my wife Dorothy came along. Yet another story for another book...

Aunt Ella began inviting me to their home in Essex for every weekend *exeat*—we had three each term. I would take the train from Epsom Downs to Paddington station right after school wound up on Friday afternoon, board the Bakerloo line tube to Oxford Circus, surface at the very centre of the teeming city, and follow her directions to the TB clinic only a block north of the tube station. I managed to get lost the first three visits: geography was never my greatest strength—and remember I was a fourteen-year-old boy getting my very first sights of London in its glory.

Auntie was often kept busy well into the evening because tuberculosis was still rampant, so Flo the tea lady would keep me supplied with sardine-and-tomato sandwiches and cream-filled doughnuts in one of the unoccupied offices. I knew to bring a book to read, every so often spying Aunt Ella bustle-bustle-bustling from room to room, offering high-pitched nonstop chuckles to her junior staff as she went about her business. What a role model she was for one who had so recently resolved to enter the caring professions, like so many of my kin.

Sometimes Auntie would introduce me to her staff, even have me join her on patient rounds, but she rarely had time for more than a fleeting visit. She knew I was set to go to medical school, and she was the first person to drum into me how much I could learn from nurses that would hold me in good stead in my chosen career. These were the days when there were many new TB drugs being developed, and Aunt Ella was responsible for early clinical trials of their effects—good and bad. It was less than twenty years since PAS—para-aminosalicylic acid—had been tested against the mycobacterium that caused the infection. It would be many years more before I realized just how painstaking these studies had to be, and how much depended on precise record keeping. Every so often a doctor would appear and Aunt Ella would drop everything to bring him (always *him*) up-to-date. But it was my auntie—that pretty, giggly, brilliant nurse from the Rhondda Valley—who ran the show.

Thank you for shining your light on the world, Aunt Ella, for saving so many lives, for teaching me the art of healing, and for being my second mum.

CHAPTER 6

The Nurses Who Cared for Us

My sister Mary was my first nurse teacher, but she wasn't the first nurse to come into my life. That would have been Nurse Lumney, the midwife who delivered me around dusk on February 23, 1942, after I'd spent my third trimester inside Mummy flipping somersaults and fattening up over Christmas. I've no idea how long she laboured over me, but I hope it was mercifully quick, me being her fourth. My father had brought Nurse Lumney all the way down from Bart's to our North Devon village of High Bickington, where he ran his rural practice. She had delivered my sisters Mary and Jane, too, travelling back and forth from the City of London each time—a full day's journey each way in those days.

Why Nurse Lumney? Couldn't my father, doctor to half of North Devon, locate a single midwife to whom he could entrust Mummy's confinements? I only found out years later that this lady was an old flame of his—and that she stayed on with us for several weeks after each birth. What Mummy thought of these arrangement I never found out. But my immediate postnatal memory—buried in there somewhere—is of my father circumcising me on our kitchen table, which served as his makeshift operating slab. No local anaesthetic of course—it was thought back then that the nerves of babies, boy ones anyway, weren't yet mature enough to feel the knife (wrong!). Nurse Lumney's embrace was my first awareness of the ancient comfort that nurses offer by instinct. It carried me through my father's brutal ceremony of foreskin lopping to my reunion with the succour of Mummy's breast. Her gazings and cooings finally calmed me from the paroxysms of birth and my severed willy.

Then came that lovely young woman whom I call *Nurse Fragrance*. When I was growing up in the forties, almost all children ran the gauntlet of T's and A's—tonsillectomy and adenoidectomy. We know now it's a largely unnecessary and dangerous procedure, which was performed mostly by family practitioners with minimal training in surgery. Let alone in how many droplets of ether to drip onto the mask about to smother my six-year-old self. (Thank the stars that my equally untrained doctor-dad was long gone out of my life by then). The doctor's sole task was to slice at lightning speed through those tonsillar and adenoidal beauties lodged well back in a suitably relaxed throat, while the nurse's exacting role (some would say far more so) was to pacify me with enough "there, theres" and oh-so-gentle "nice and still nows" to speed up the doctor's work.

I don't have a clear vision of Nurse Fragrance's face as she cuddled me before the dread mask descended upon my terrified countenance, but the aroma of her scent will be with me forever. Should I get a whiff of that same delicate perfume today it would transport me back seventy and more years. My first awareness on reviving from the ether was the appalling pain in my throat. *NPO (nil by mouth)* for four hours after anesthesia may have been the strict rule, but I was having none of it. One hoarse and agonized screech summoned the scented loveliness to my bedside. Surely she knew ice cream to be strictly banned? But it took only a couple of delicious pain-banishing frozen chocolate mouthfuls to hush my screams. An utterly delicious minute later I barfed the whole concoction onto my blanket, accompanied by globular strings of mucus and congealed blood.

I'll love you forever, Nurse Fragrance—and I'm awfully sorry I gave you that stinky mess to clean up.

When I finally grew to be on the delivery end of a knife or forceps, I quickly found out that my best chance for a swift and successful procedure on any small child—inserting a lumbar puncture needle or getting an IV in place in a miniscule vein—relied solely on the skill of my nursing assistant. Securing a rambunctious toddler in her arms, while always keeping the target exposed to my hovering needle, is a consummate art.

I met my Aunt Muriel soon after I went to St. Peter's primary school at aged seven. She wasn't really family but I always called her Auntie. She often came to visit her sister Margaret, my best mate Mike's mum, and the two sisters were like identical twins—small and energetic, with short dark hair and rosy English complexions.

My sister Mary told me later that Muriel was the night nurse in charge of the surgery ward where Mummy died. Mary carried a lifelong grudge towards her because she wouldn't let her in to see our mother on her death bed. This was January 1955, and Mary had turned eighteen the previous Christmas Day, so she was already accepted for nursing training at Bart's. But Aunt Muriel clearly thought it better for us children to remember Mummy the way she had always been—*Tigger* to her college friends—*Pooh, Piglet,* and *Eeyore*—for her bouncy ebullient ways. She judged it would do more harm than good to expose us children to the sight of Mummy in a pre-death morphine coma after the "open-and-shut" surgery for hopelessly inoperable cancer throughout her abdomen.

Today Muriel might have made a different decision, but there wasn't, and still isn't, a clear protocol in these matters, and the doctors would have left it solely to the nurses to decide what was best. Knowing Aunt Muriel as a gentle, caring nurse, I have no doubt she gave Mummy, in her last decidely "unbouncy" days, all the loving care that she had within her.

Early in my medical internship at Barts, Aunt Ella and Uncle Roger retired back to their roots in the Rhondda Valley where they both had family. But they had barely time to enjoy their leisure. First, Uncle Roger suffered a massive stroke that left him mute. He lasted only three months before he quietly stopped breathing. Then within months, Aunt Ella developed an inoperable abdominal cancer—an echo of my mother's. She lingered on for several weeks in coma, due to spread of the cancer to her brain abetted by escalating doses of morphine. I couldn't get away for several weeks from my internship at Bart's, but I finally drove the 150 miles from my Tufnell Park flat in north London to Cardiff General Hospital. I checked in at the front desk and the sister in charge at once poked her head out of her office.

"Come on in. We've been expecting you. We knew it was hard for you to get away."

Her quiet voice calmed my nerves after the jangle of four hours highway driving. She indicated the chair next to her own behind her desk.

"John, is it? I'm so sorry we're meeting in these sad circumstances. Your auntie is comfy—we just upped her morphine dose—but she may not know you." She paused and held my look. "I don't think it will be long."

She led me back out to the ward and down the corridor to a single room. "I'll leave you to have some privacy. Call me if you need to."

I felt my sobs well up—far from the first time a nurse's tenderness had evoked tears in me. I edged open the door to Aunt Ella's private room. My auntie was lying mute and immobile, in such unhappy contrast to her usual vivacity; she was surely unaware of my presence at her bedside. Her breaths were coming only periodically, with a long intake followed by no breath at all for several seconds, then another long gasp. My internship on Bart's oncology wards had taught me to call this unmistakable pattern Cheyne-Stokes breathing—sometimes called periodic. A sure sign a person is not long for this world.

I pulled up a chair beside her, grasped her hand, murmured, "Hallo, Auntie. It's John. Sorry I couldn't get here sooner." As I watched, she released one more breath, which proved to be her last one on Earth. It was as if she had been waiting for me.

Forward a quarter-century to 1992: my father's deathbed. He had outlived Mummy by fifty years, then died quickly from acute monoblastic leukemia—a rare illness in the old.

He had himself admitted to the Freeman Hospital in New-castle-on-Tyne, where he challenged his doctors with tests of his own concoction. My sister Jane phoned me at work at Shands Hospital in Florida where I was at work on the pediatric wards.

"They don't give him long," she told me. "Maybe a few weeks. But he's determined to receive chemotherapy."

I shuddered at the thought of my eighty-seven-year-old dad suffering through the rigours of intensive chemotherapy, whose horrid toxicities I witnessed every day. I stood stock still in the nurses' station of the Shands pediatric ICU, weeping for the unresolved issues between us, grieving the bitter way our patchwork fifty-year relationship had ended in this final and total disconnection. Ayman, a second-year fellow in our oncology department, stood silently beside me. Gifted with an innate flare for empathy, he wrapped his comforting Syrian arms around me, then took over my attending duties without a pause while I flew home to England.

Before boarding my plane I put in a last call to my father's hospital ward, only to learn that he had died six hours earlier, lulled in the arms of merciful narcosis. After the funeral I drove to Newcastle to visit the ward in the Freeman Hospital where he had died. Judith, my father's nurse for his last night on earth, greeted me. She and I sat together in the visitor's lounge next to the Muslim prayer room, looking out on the distant River Tyne as she told me the story of the short time she had spent nursing my doctor-dad. How she had sat with him through his last hours, topping up his merciful infusion of narcotic.

"My shift was over, but I asked if I could stay on with him. I knew it wouldn't be long. Your dad was trying to hide his terror behind all that belligerence. He'd scared off the interns by trying to write his own medical orders, but he knew he wasn't about to push me around. Doctor Phillips, his consultant, let me manage the morphine, but it took a good bit to get him settled."

It was comforting to sit beside this competent and mer-ciful young woman. To picture her sitting close beside my dad as he released his final breath and died.

CHAPTER 7

Touching

I think often of those nurses who made such close connections with my beloved family members. Beside the bedsides of the dying the barriers have to come down-down-down: it's no place for "professional distance." Nurses learn early to lay on their hands, together with their other senses—seeing, listening, attending—in ways that defy any scientific measure. They seem to bring to their work better instincts than doctors, are quicker to learn and accept—hopefully to welcome and nurture—intimacy with their patients. Bedpans and bed baths inevitably create this climate, which certainly helps; how many bedpans did I clean in my forty-seven years? Yet the best nurses I have known see keeping a helpless invalid clean and comfy as a simple labour of love.

We doctors rarely allow ourselves such close bonds—we have no Bedside Manner 101 manual. Intimate connections between doctors and those we care for are just beginning to be encouraged, even embraced. For nurses this empathy is as ancient as their profession. They spend a lot of time alone with their patients—as partner and as witness. Medicine is certainly full of beautiful words and phrases—and thank god for them—but those very words can sometimes reinforce that professional distance between us and those we care for. Many nurses seem to develop an unspoken communication, as though they and their charges are journeying together between sickness and health.

Though I had little natural aptitude for the biomedical sciences—too little, I thought at first, for the calling I had chosen—it was through nurses that I came to know I was no impostor in my profession. To recognize early that I was contributing something *substantial* when I slowed down enough to sit, first, at those bedsides—then, as my confidence grew, on their beds—to simply bear witness and listen.

The art of touch is perhaps what most distinguishes nurses from doctors. Few nurses hesitate to touch their patients; perhaps that's what they do the very best. A necessity, of course, when you spend much of your day bathing and turning and propping up and easing down. But the nurses I have known mostly seemed to take joy in making these essential touches a *therapeutic* act rather than the *diagnostic* one the doctor's touch so often is. It was nurses who taught me it was just fine—actually vital—to make touch an act of healing.

That word *touch*—physical, emotional, spiritual—is the one Louise Erdrich chose to use in her novel *Love Medicine* to describe an act of healing. Chippewa Lipsha Morrisey declares his shamanic power in this way:

"*I know tricks of the mind and body inside out without ever having trained for it, because I got the touch. It's a thing you got to be born with...The medicine flows out of me. The Touch.*"

But the notion runs deep in us doctors that "getting too close" (*what does that even mean?*) will hamper our clinical judgment. So we imbibe early on the lesson that we must keep our professional distance. Yet almost all of us have ourselves savored the rapture of soul-to-soul love. We were blessed with it within minutes of our earthly life when we were lifted into the arms of the one who had just birthed us. And we instinctively bestowed our mother's love right back, as the two of us healed together from the jarring paroxysms of birth. The evolutionary anthropologist Ellen Dissanayake highlights in her book *Art and Intimacy* this mutual duet between a mother and her newborn—at once *visual, vocal, performative* and *tactile*. Such intimate connection is a *human universal*; what a deep blessing that our nurses get to put these instincts to work their every working day.

We doctors make diagnoses, and prognoses, and write our endless orders; but it's our nurses who carry them through. Ultimately, they run the show. As I was building my career as a medical scientist-researcher, I got to learn the niceties of every new cancer drug as it came down the line; very soon I was devoting all my time to designing and drawing up new protocols. But it was always the nurses who administered those drug protocols at the bedside—and sought to lessen the horrendous side effects for their woeful recipients. Who but a nurse cleans up sputum, vomit, urine, faeces, blood from a helpless patient? Much of a nurse's work is mopping up the messes that these often powerless bodies create. I have never brushed another adult's teeth, nor given them a bed bath. Physical stamina and a thick skin are indispensable to doing such work well.

Only once did I get to mop up a patient's shit. It was Jim, a charge nurse on the pediatric ward, who put me to work. He pressed me to take a break as I made my doctor rounds to get close and personal with my seventeen-year-old patient. Stevie had Duchenne's muscular dystrophy; he had not one functional muscle below his clavicles. When I arrived at his room, Jim was cleaning the bubbles and squirts coming out of Stevie's bottom, in preparation for returning his bed to its wrinkle-free purity.

"Come on, John, time to get your hands dirty!"

No female nurse in my working lifetime had ever issued such a summons. Stevie, long used to total dependency on others for these tasks, grinned at Jim's jokey tone and at the notion of his doctor cleaning his bottom. It was a memorable first for me, though it was an almost hourly task for his nurse. To get to a place not just of acceptance but of active support for a helpless patient's shame and misery, nurses must deal with their own lifelong repulsions. Only in this way can they help their patient retain their own dignity. Jim taught me not only this essential lesson, but also, not incidentally, the art of perfecting a hospital corner as we made up Stevie's bed together.

How often do nurses wash their hands in a given 8- or 10- or 12-hour shift? I overheard two nurses in the sluice compare the effectiveness of lanolin and Vaseline for protecting their hands from painful rawness. I have seen nurses at the start of their shifts—freshly showered and vibrant—and those same nurses twelve hours later—rumpled and exhausted and all set to chuck it in for a job in the secretary pool. But they don't get to graduate from being in close quarters with their patients, the way many doctors open up greater and greater distances as they graduate up the ranks of intern to senior resident to fellow to attending physician. And nowadays the telephone seems to be replacing the stethoscope as our favourite diagnostic tool.

This laying on of hands on our patients is an ancient tradition, both religious and secular. It is an intimate act that evokes physical, emotional and spiritual healing. The most vivid instance of loving touch I ever witnessed was after I became a pediatric palliative care director. One of our hospice nurses, Cendra, was at the bedside of a thirteen-year-old girl who was close to death. She had had no family visits since her admission; on the rare occasions we managed to reach her parents they told us they just couldn't deal with the whole thing. The girl was crying constantly from pain and fear, so late that last evening Cendra climbed into her bed and held her in her arms until she died at five o'clock the next morning.

CHAPTER 8

Midder

If I ever doubted how much nurses had to teach me, it took a day and a night of midwifery to set me straight. It was 1963: my medical student training month at the North Middlesex Hospital—and a time of rapture. For my first couple of days the world-weary senior house officer, Dave Shand, tossed me odd crumbs of obstetrical lore, even as he was hefting yet another pregnant lady's legs up into the stirrups for the endless pelvic exams considered vital to modern antenatal care. It took only three days before he was leaving me to the tender care of those motherly midwives. Two generations ago during my callow med student years, Britain's midwives were still our primary mentors in the art of birthing babies. They worked largely in these outlying community hospitals and dedicated childbirth centres, simply because that was where most mothers birthed their babies.

The profession dates back to Ancient Egypt and Greece, and the word *midwife* goes back at least to 1300 AD, meaning a woman who "stands with" a birthing woman and her baby. For millennia, women sat supported by birthing chairs as their babies obeyed the natural impulse of gravity. Though Aristotle admired midwives for their wisdom and dedication, nowadays the whole thing has been almost taken over by hospital-based obstetricians. Many of them are men, and they seem to think of pregnancy as a pathological condition. How did we men get in on this quintessentially female act—once we'd played out our very brief part in a baby's procreation?

I watched my very first delivery over a seasoned midwife's shoulder. As the product of a boys-only boarding school, I was quite unversed in the ways of the world, and it took me a dizzying few days to recover from my first full-frontal view of the female form in its gravid state. It seemed there was no need to seek permission to attend these intimate encounters with such womanly beauty. But thank the stars my face was hidden behind a mask—at twenty-two I looked seventeen; if I had grown up in the United States I would have been carded until I was thirty. The midwife started talking to me without turning her head.

"My name's Ellen, by the way. What's yours?"

"John."

"This will be Mrs. Stafford's sixth baby, John, and her previous five all went to term. You'll see in her chart that she's G5 P5—that's midder-speak for *gravida five, para five.* Which means she's been pregnant five times and has had healthy babies each time. No miscarriages, right, Polly?"

Polly was too preoccupied to answer, already up in the stirrups and starting to push.

"Polly, John's a medical student here to learn Midder. You're pretty used to that by now, right? Okay if he calls you Polly?"

More groans from Polly: was that assent—or simply insistence to get the thing done? Liquid was running down the inside of her thighs—amniotic fluid, urine, or honest sweat? Had I missed her water breaking? I had the hazy idea that this was how the baby announced its imminent arrival—and if this was number six, it shouldn't take long. I was tense with excitement, about to witness my first birth from a front-row seat. Polly was grunting and pushing under Ellen's guidance, now winging a string of colorful curses her old man's way for once more knocking her up. I wondered briefly where he was—in the pub with his mates? No doubt he enjoyed the conception end of things a whole lot more than the delivery.

The baby came fast, pink and plump, squirming and yowling by the time Ellen got to suction her mouth and nose. She passed her over to me to lay on the scales by the bed.

"Weight? Apgar score?"

I had no time to reflect on this moment of holding my very first newborn baby in my arms as my mind crashed through the pages of *The OBG (Obstetrics and Gynecology) Yearbook.* Hallelujah, that word *Apgar* rang a faint bell. Our obstetrics prof. was my favorite so I had clung onto a few pearls. *Heart rate, respirations, muscle tone, response, colour.... That's it!*

"Er. . .seven pounds, eight. . .no, ten ounces." Ellen looked over to check my accuracy as I grabbed my stethoscope. "Er. . .pink-appearing = 2, lusty cry = 2, um. . .good tone = 2." I grasped the tiny, slippery hands and drew her upwards. "Flexes actively = 2..." I placed my stethoscope in the region of the baby's swollen left nipple, that of a young woman's. "Er. . .can't count her heart rate, too fast..."

Ellen handed me a warm towel and unrolled a miniscule blanket from the radiator.

"Quick, get her wrapped up, we don't want her catching her death now, do we? And any heart rate over a hundred scores a 2 as well. So what've you got?"

The baby girl's eyes were shut tight. I gazed entranced at her tiny pinkness.

"*Apgar*, John?" I sensed mild irritation in her querying, but mostly amusement.

"Er, *Apgar 10*. That's great!"

"Ever held a newborn before?"

"No, it's my first time."

"Okay, Polly's turn. Let's try the baby's suck."

Ellen lifted the swaddled bundle out of my arms, laid her beside the already slumbering Polly, loosened the gown to expose her breast, and guided the swollen nipple towards the baby's mouth. She rooted briefly, latched on, then she too was fast asleep.

My exhilaration amounted to awe—to be present at the birth and first breath of this perfect human creature. The outcome of one brief act of coupling, and forty weeks of molding each autonomous organ and appendage. My mind was taking flight: *Wow, what a work of art…* Then I caught Ellen grinning at me. This may have been bread-and-butter to her, but it just could be she was enjoying my rapture.

"You did well, John. We'll make an obstetrician of you yet. Who knows, maybe a midwife!"

And within days I found myself the sole attendant on my very own *accouchement* stool, giving me a front-row seat as yet another newborn slipped and slid his way into our world. He needed minimal guidance from me, clearly knew how to get the job done—like he'd been here before. … My month passed in a whirl of deliveries at all hours of day and night, with just the occasional prenatal and postnatal check-up sessions by Dave Shand thrown in. I even managed to fit in a brief but torrid encounter with a student midwife. Waking up beside her to the shrill of my early-morning beeper, I was grabbing my clothes when she stirred and the whole sheet slipped to the floor. I felt a strong desire to hop right back into bed.

"Maybe I'll ignore that, tell them I never got the call—battery must have been flat."

She giggled. "You'd think you'd be turned off after all those deliveries."

"No way that's going to happen."

"That's good."

She grinned again, hauled up the bedclothes, and was fast asleep again before I was out the door.

My midwife mentors were quickly leaving me to *stand with* the birthing mum. See one, do one, teach one was clearly their motto—though the about-to-be mums had no notion of my brand new exposure to this blessed art. Most of my learning seemed to take place between noon on Fridays and six on Saturday mornings. I figured this was the time babies mostly chose to alight on our earth, no doubt favoring the idea of starting out life on a weekend. This was the sixties, and babies were largely left to tick to their own biological clocks, and they were in no hurry to leave the blissful comfort of their watery wombs.

Today's obstetricians respond to such tardiness by infusing the mum-to-be with Pitocin to speed up her contractions, if not whisking her straight off to the operating room for a C-section. In the USA, the C-section rate was 5% in 1970 but today accounts for almost one third of births. The babies let everyone in hearing distance know just what they think of this rough and ready treatment. It's no surprise that their universal greeting to the world is to scream loud and long—indeed, the absence of any such fury causes consternation all round. Some of us probably spend our lives scarred by such traumatic beginnings.

Friday evenings we medical students had established a longstanding habit of hitting the pubs surrounding Bart's Hospital and its nearby med school. But this idyllic month found me each Friday evening perched on a low accouchement stool between the legs of a multiparous mum. My accustomed place in the breach, with the birthing stool's casters swiveling freely on their axis, raised the distinct possibility of my pivoting backwards or—much worse—forwards. The midwives showed up less and less often to check on me—as much because of the "nothing-to-it" multiparity of most of our charges as any great faith in my skills. It was quite customary for the mother or sister of mum-to-be to be entertaining three or four of her toddlers in the waiting room. Even more astounding, these seasoned women seemed to trust me in my crucial role.

I cherished it that so few women ever questioned my credentials or showed the slightest embarrassment at baring their bodies before me. And faced with such awesome responsibilities for bringing forth new life, I quickly left behind my adolescent self-doubt and found myself taking charge. In one twenty-four-hour spell I delivered three babies, snatching brief in-between catnaps on the couch in the midwives' lounge. I was on a lasting high, fueled by surges of endorphins at my newfound skills. My joy amounted to ecstasy as I became the attendant at this mysterious act of birth. I didn't think of it then, but I now see this God-given ritual—the very origin of our human race—as a sacred mystery as momentous as the moment of our death.

Once I had the thing down I eased into the role of witness, and intervened just enough to guide the baby's progress when absolutely needed. Which wasn't often: this divine and natural act is the rite of passage for every one of us sentient beings. So I spent more and more time getting to know these awesome women, doing all I could to relieve their physical pain so that they too could capture some of the magic of it. Most of these new, or not so new, mothers were either too exhausted or too used to these delivery room encounters to have much resource for joy. But even those who had been through the laborious business as much as a dozen times responded to the moment of delivery with breathless delight at uniting with their new offspring. For almost half our human race, this must be life's ultimate accomplishment.

For me, too, the crowning point was my all too brief acquaintance with these sacred new beings. How apt that the moment the head appears at the vulval entrance to announce the baby's imminent arrival is dubbed the *crowning*. With the cutting of the cord, and with their first strident cry out into the world, these slippery, bloody creatures, faces temporarily squished and scalps misshapen from their arduous trip down the birth canal, proclaimed their arrival. Their first protests behind them, they were *here*, and they were *now*. As yet untouched by the distresses of the world, they were free of all judgment or remorse.

But by no means is every birth a joyful experience. It can be an immense and heart-wrenching problem to judge if a newborn babe is really ready to join us. I got a call one night from the duty midwife to scuttle to the Labor & Delivery suite *asap*.

"Anne here, John. The ambulance just brought this young girl in. She started bleeding early this evening and it looks like she's about to deliver. She claims she didn't know she was pregnant, but she must be well along judging by the looks of things. There's no family with her."

By the time I made it to the unit, Anne was completing a pelvic exam on mum-to-be. She looked about fourteen, maybe less, and terrified.

"I estimate she's around thirty weeks," Anne told me quietly. "No antenatal care at all. The baby's alive, but in a lot of distress. Heartbeat over two hundred, and very weak. It'll be touch and go."

Ten minutes later, Mum pushed out her son with barely a whimper. He was dusky blue and looked lifeless. He weighed about two pounds, if that. Anne passed him into my waiting arms. The new mum swiftly subsided back into an exhausted sleep, so she didn't have to witness everything that was happening. I rushed the small bundle of limpness over to the exam table, listened for a heartbeat as Anne struggled to fasten an oxygen mask over his titchy face. The heartbeat was there but thready, and far too fast to count. I suctioned the little mite as gently as I could; he responded with the feeblest of cries and a couple of uncertain gasps, but with no lessening of his duskiness.

I lifted the mask up an inch to offer him my finger, but he had no power, nor even apparent instinct, to suck. He needed an immediate intravenous infusion of fluids if we were going to restore him to life, but I couldn't imagine getting a needle into his almost non-existent veins. It felt like an exercise in total futility, but surely we couldn't just let him die... could we?

Anne interrupted my pondering. "Let's get him weighed."

We unwrapped him briefly from his cozy covers and laid him on the infant scales.

"Two pounds, four ounces," she read off. "Can't remember having one this size who made it. You'd better phone Dave Shand."

Her soft tones were suddenly comforting. I glanced up at her. "You're right. Thanks."

"And how about having Mum recover in a private room in the pediatric ward? After all, she's barely fourteen years old, and she needs the kind of care that those peds nurses can give her."

"Right. Right. Thanks."

CHAPTER 9

Me? A Surgeon?

I was never cut out to master the art of surgery. My father was a natural with a scalpel and a needle, and with a paintbrush too, but he passed none of those skills down to me. Fortunately I had no inclination to learn either the art or the techniques of these skills. There was, however, one glorious morning when I could take pride in my skills with a surgical instrument. And there being no surgeon to guide me, it was a nurse who proved my sole mentor.

It was the early summer of 1969 and I was making rounds in Jenny Lind Children's Hospital in Norwich, in Britain's Fen country. It was the end of my day as a new pediatric resident, and the night nurse was introducing me to the patients who'd been admitted that afternoon. She paused to ruffle a toddler's curls.

"One of your OR cases for the morning, doctor. Circs."

"Circs?" The word bewildered me. "Ah, *circs!*" I tried to cover my confusion. "But I thought they did those at birth?"

"Oh, they're much choosier nowadays. Only do the essential ones. Phimosis, that kind of thing."

I had only the vaguest notion what "phimosis" was— something to do with a toddler's foreskin being too tight to pee out a healthy stream? Nevertheless, at eight sharp next morning I found my way to the operating theatre. It took me only a glance around the changing room to confirm I was the only possible surgeon in sight. I eyed my scrubbed-in nurse partner as she splashed large blobs of Betadine onto the tiny penis of the first case for the morning's surgery. It was one of the toddlers I had cast my eyes over the evening before at the night nurse's prompting: she had pointed out gently that I should check over each of what to proved to be my six "cases," to make doubly sure they were fit and well enough for tomorrow's ordeal. I noted with some relief that he was now fast in the land of nod, which led me to glace briefly at the older man sitting at the head of my operating table. He was idly twiddling some of the nobs on his gas machine as he undolded the newspaper in his lap.

Is he going to be inspecting my handiwork? And is he going to know when to wake my patient up?

My nurse-partner finished wrapping my minute operating field in sterile green and handed me a miniscule scalpel. She broke the silence that had been gathering about us as though in church.

"Probably didn't warn you to expect this. Fear not, I've trained a few resident doctors in my time."

Nurses teaching doctors? Is this even legal?

I sensed the smirk beneath the mask, spotted wisps of grey hair escaping from beneath her cap. No names had been exchanged, but I was all set to follow her directions to the tee.

"First, you're going to slit open his foreskin, doctor. Right here. Now push back with your fingers, so just his little knob is sticking out. The business end, doctor, you might call it."

Did I detect a faint irony as she pronounced that word *doctor*? Not just once but twice? I snipped tentatively as directed along the tiny pecker. There was a disturbing intimacy about this whole scene—this motherly nurse, this little boy's tiny appendage, and *moi*. Was I cutting into the little mite's future pleasure?

"Now draw his foreskin over the top of this thingy."

I quickly complied as she plucked a diminutive plastic ring from her arsenal of surgical gadgets—the thingy. Her oh-so-competent hands guided my own oh-so-hesitant ones.

"Now tie this ligature round to staunch the blood when you chop it off."

With no idea where I was headed, I could only assume she meant just the foreskin, not the whole organ. Sweat was trickling freely down my forehead as I pulled the nylon suture taut. She handed me a pair of miniature surgical scissors. I could barely squeeze my finger and thumb tip through the loops.

"Now, the *coup de grace*! Lop it off!"

The tiny integument plopped into her waiting basin. She cocooned the remaining intact member in bandages, leaving a single centimeter sticking out.

"Well done, doctor!"

"Can't claim much credit."

"Nonsense! See one, do one, teach one. You'll be a pro in no time."

This time the irony came through clearly. I was moved to both laughter and tears. Yet sure enough, the remaining circumcisions got steadily easier; by morning's end I felt like I could teach the whole thing without guidance. What the mums of these toddlers would think remained to be seen.

I never inquired into the legality of this whole business, but we were buried deep in the fens and grasslands of rural Norfolk—and I had no reason to doubt this nurse's claim that she had taught a whole generation of medical interns before me.

CHAPTER 10

Ministering Angel

But I wasn't destined to totally avoid the role of surgeon. We took turns covering Jenny Lind's Accident & Emergency (A&E) department, dealing with cuts and grazes, dislodged joints and bowed bones, sustained in playgrounds and backyards and from bicycle wipeouts. Rosemary had been the nurse in charge there for twenty years, and she had learned her many skills way back from her own nurse-mentor.

The first thing she taught me was the not-so-gentle art of straightening greenstick fractures, named for the "greener" nature of children's bones. These bones were like healthy new-grown saplings. Mostly all that was needed was a plaster cast and the bent bone aligned flawlessly into its pristine shape. Applying the plaster of Paris was a marvelously sloppy task. Rosemary would dip lengths of cotton bandage into the goop and hand me the sticky end. Then she would guide my hands as I wound it just tight enough around a wriggling shin or forearm before it set too hard and was rendered worthless. A happening I was guilty of more than once early on, but Rosemary remained a steadfast source of patience and praise.

The younger children saw no reason to restrain their feelings and would offer up a cacophony of screams and howls—more from fear than from pain. They had yet to learn the inhibition that muted their older brothers and sisters. But once the deed was done these toddlers were quickly chattering and laughing as if nothing bad had ever afflicted them. Meanwhile, I learned to disguise the roughness and puckers of my plaster casts with cartoons in unheard-of patterns, thanks to Rosemary's store of colored pens. Suddenly I was an artist. And unlike grown-ups, who judge a surgeon's skill from the fineness of their scar, all these children exacted from me was my signature. Another treaty signed in poster paint. How many years had it been since I'd had such fun?

After my several vain attempts to draw blood samples from the veins that lay under the pudgy backs of toddler hands, Rosemary taught me the astounding trick of collecting these samples through a baby's "soft spot"—the anterior fontanelle overlying the sagittal sinus that lies just beneath the calvarium of the skull.

"Just place your needle flat and point it straight back," she guided me. "Then drop it down a fraction. There, see?" To my astonishment blood was flowing under gentle pressure straight into my syringe. "Now swing the baby upright and keep pressing on your puncture for a minute. There, you see how easy that is." She added as an afterthought, "the docs aren't too much in favour of it till they come to realize just how safe and easy it is."

But by six months or so the baby's fontanelle is closed up and no longer accessible. So after that, when it came to starting IVs on young ones who needed antibiotics or a blood transfusion, the back of the hand was essentially the only option. Rosemary had an instinct for just where a tiny vein would allow access, as she managed to keep a firm grip on a sweaty wrist and calm the little one with motherly coddling and lullabying. But it was when it came to undertaking lumbar punctures on these young ones that I became eternally grateful to her. There was no mistaking the telltale signs of meningitis—raging fever, delirium, and a neck too rigid to flex forward one iota. I had become adept enough at performing LPs on more or less cooperative adults, but those toddlers were a whole other kettle of fish. The precious secret lay in Rosemary's ability to curl the child securely in her arms on his side so that his supple lumbar spine was spread out in such a way as to make access to my target—the subarachnoid space—a no-brainer. It became a quick and simple matter to capture my precious sample of cerebrospinal fluid and whisk it off to the lab for diagnosis.

Rosemary was always infinitely tactful towards my easily bruised ego, just as she must have been towards a generation of budding pediatricians. I went all out to perform my tasks as adeptly as possible, hating the task of wounding these fragile beings, and certain that the traumas I was inflicting upon them they would carry to their graves. As indeed would I.

But the rites of passage had to be marked if I was to become seasoned as a children's doctor. Those adult cancer patients on Dalziel and Annie Zunz wards back at Bart's mostly went along with our terrible and largely experimental treatments—therapies that in those days only delayed the inevitable outcome. But did the end—that of learning a fraction more about our highly experimental chemo regimens—justify these means? So how much harder for children, who had no legal right to refuse these awful treatments. If ethical issues are tough in the world of adult medicine, how much more so when it comes to young ones. It was thanks to those nurses, together with children's natural resilience, that my patients' complaints were mostly short lived.

It was a month after my arrival at Jenny Lind that I met my first child with cancer. Audrey was eight years old and had widespread neuroblastoma, a cancer I had never encountered in my year on Bart's adult oncology wards. This was 1969 and treatment for children with the new chemo drugs was still in its infancy; so it turned out my medical bosses had never ever treated a child with cancer. I was still very new on the block, and my seniors had a lot of trouble letting me loose on their patients with these, to them, totally unfamiliar chemo drugs.

But the ward sister backed me up when I explained what they could expect and how we would manage the side effects that would inevitably crop up. The hospital's senior doctor, John Quinton, had had very little time to get to know me, let alone put any trust in my abilities, but he and that ward sister went back a long way. He reluctantly agreed to my treating Audrey with chemotherapy. Within weeks the little girl had achieved a complete response to the regimen I had both prescribed and administered. She was soon running around the outpatient clinic with no signs of the horrid disease that had ravaged her body just a short while before. The nurses were as delighted as me to witness this apparent miracle.

This state of affairs persisted for a blissful eight months; then early one morning Rosemary phoned me from Accident & Emergency.

"Audrey's here with her mum, John. She doesn't look well at all, and she's complaining of a lot of pain in her tummy and her right leg."

My heart sank. I had known this was almost certain to happen sooner or later, but I had tried hard to put the likelihood out of my mind as the last happy months had passed and Audrey had seemed in such robust health.

"John, I know how attached you've become to her, and how hard this will be for you. I'm going to call Dr. Quinton to help you deal with things. And I've got some help today, so I can stay with her."

And with me please. I'm going to want someone holding my hand, too.

The telltale signs were all too clear. Audrey lay quietly on the exam table, legs tucked up as if trying to keep them halfway comfy. Though she was running a fever of 101, there was no sign of any infection. I felt the hardness of her liver, just as I had eight months earlier, and she flinched when I tried to bend her right knee.

"They told me in med school not to let this happen," I told Rosemary quietly once I'd finished my exam. "Keep your professional distance was the message."

"Easy to say, John. It doesn't always work that way."

"I don't know, I'm not sure if I'm cut out for this kind of work."

"That's just where you're wrong. It's the doctors who struggle to bottle up their feelings who get into trouble down the road. I've seen it a lot." I was on the point of losing it, but Rosemary must have sensed this and promptly became matter-of-fact. "I'll stay right here while you talk to Audrey's mum."

Audrey lived on for a few short weeks. Once we admitted her, the ward nurses became ministering angels to the little girl, to her parents, and to me. They encouraged me to order regular small doses of morphine for her tummy and bone pain; this proved highly effective, especially because she was eating next to nothing. I had an inkling that the opiate doses were shortening Audrey's time with us, but no one queried my prescription. Both parents and staff were relieved to see the little one relaxed and comfy. The same couple of nurses rotated her care in a private room on the ward, and I spent time at her bedside each day, mostly in the late afternoon before finishing work.

Just before the end, I got a phone call from her night nurse. "She's woken up, John. And she's pretty perky. Chatting away to her parents, though I don't think they can follow anything she's saying. I thought you'd want to know."

It was a peaceful end. I hugged the parents, and the night nurse hugged me. "That jumbled chatter—it quite often happens, you know, just before a child passes. I always think it's a comforting sign."

CHAPTER 11

Learning at Their Knees

I praise nurses I have worked with who are unafraid to speak up and put a doctor straight when they question his judgment. A Puerto Rican mother told me of a surgeon at an eminent hospital, whom she had consulted about possible surgery for her son's severe disability. The doctor talked exclusively to his nurse, never addressing a word to her. It was left entirely to the nurse, who also happened to be Hispanic, to translate everything into Spanish that the man had said, because the mother had no chance to tell the doctor she understood his every word. He simply told his nurse, "No way I'm going to touch this case," which the nurse gently translated to the mother as, "The doctor's sorry, but he doesn't feel he can operate on your baby." The doctor gave no explanation whatsoever, even to his nurse, for why he wouldn't even attempt the operation. But by this time the nurse knew Mum spoke fluent English, and she didn't hesitate to let the surgeon know that this mother had understood every word he had uttered.

Today, the symbolism of the starched, pristine, maidenly nurse's uniform and cap of my student days have completely vanished, along with the teaching—Oh god, good riddance!—that the doctor is always right and must be obeyed implicitly. A nurse who doesn't challenge the most senior doctor on the block for what that nurse considers a wrong decision, or a wrongly written prescription, is falling short of her duty. So thank goodness more and more are screwing their courage to the sticking post when they witness doctors explaining an illness or its treatment in complex language clearly—perhaps even intentionally—beyond their patient's grasp. These nurses may or may not at once take issue with the doctor's language, but they won't hesitate to linger behind, sit down by the bed, and explain it in everyday language. While never talking down to the patient.

Too often we doctors are only a presence in a patient's doorway, perching briefly to probe a chest or abdomen. Maintaining a healthy professional distance may be good in theory, but how can you possibly learn where to draw that line? *What does such a directive even mean?* Meanwhile, nurses are a constant bedside presence—assessing, calming, hand-holding, listening, caring, explaining, mentoring, coordinating everything that is going on. As the distinguished poet and nurse Courtney Davis says in her book, *Between the Lines*, saving our patients' lives is *not* the primary task; caring, listening, advocating *are*.

Patients' suffering is largely in our nurses' hands. It is they who give the injections, start, and restart, the IVs, pass catheters, suction airways, clean wounds. And often many times a day. No one taught me how to offer the simple comfort measures to a helplessly ill patient of bathing, shaving, turning, and back rubbing. I cannot imagine teaching a spouse, a parent, and most especially a child patient, how to suction their tracheostomy tube. Yet this may well be a vital part of a nurse's daily work.

The best nurses are as good as doctors at diagnosing what's wrong with a patient—as if they develop an instinct over the years to sniff out trouble as soon as they enter the room. They are party to those patient secrets that they know never to share with me. And their technical competence is awe-inspiring. They seem totally in sync with every labelled bag and bottle and spaghetti strand of tubing—a complexity I find daunting. Almost every patient in an intensive care unit is on life support of some kind. Those ICU nurses understand up and down and inside out machines that I had never been trained on.

Most of what I knew about nurses early on had to do with the immense emotional support they offered; I gave little thought to the wealth of scientific training they receive and technical competence they develop. When I was an intern in England it was still my job to draw all the bloods and start all the IVs; today, nurses have largely subsumed these tasks. And it was they who pushed for implanted IV access ports for chemo infusions, which up till then would wreck every available vein. Did a doctor think of this simple, but so, so compassionate, application of science and technology? No, it was a nurse!

As I moved up the ladder in my profession, it became a common sight on rounds for me to see a nurse analyze a patient's degree of hypoxia from their arterial blood gases and instantly correct it, all the while cleaning up their pee and poop. I once watched an ICU nurse prepare for a trauma victim set to arrive in her pod. She unlocked the medical supply cart to check the presence of needles of every size, alcohol pads, gauze pads, sterile saline, oxygen tubing. Then she attached suction tubing to the plastic oxygen port on the wall, before counting out the packages of artificial airways, intubation equipment, tracheostomy kits, resuscitation bag and masks of every size. She checked the packs of wire leads for heart monitoring, then made sure the monitor screen was functioning perfectly, before hanging IV bags ready to hook up to the patient for drawing blood and infusing fluids and medication. Finally, she confirmed there were adequate supplies of sheets, blankets, towels, washcloths, toothettes, sheets, and absorbent pads.

Everything seemed second nature to her as she systematically checked off her mental list; yet could I have ever mastered this complex ritual? Nurses need the kind of intense sustained focus rarely demanded of me as an intern, let alone as a professor. Yet it was those nurses who taught me the incalculable value of simply sitting and listening: "Get to know them a little," was the memorable phrase one nurse used. "You don't need to be *doing* something to your patient every minute you spend with them."

It was Florence Nightingale who challenged physicians' conviction that to give medicine, however unproven, was to do *something*, meaning everything possible. While to supply clean air, warmth, and cleanliness—the very elements of good nursing—was to do *nothing*. The nurses I have known almost always saw their primary task as caring, listening, and cheering on, rather than curing at whatever cost. They were almost always the best advocates for their patients and their families, especially when that patient or family disagreed with a physician's advice or proposed plan of action. Nurses' clarity about the best interests of their patient come directly from their constant close contact with them as *individual people*. They are not only far closer than most doctors to these sick ones, but often to their families too. And even after a decision is made to suspend life-preserving treatment, no nurse will ever withdraw loving care.

We are all potential patients. I just hope there's a good nurse there for me when it happens.

CHAPTER 12

Glaswegian Bairns

In 1972, when I moved from London to Glasgow to continue my training in Pediatrics, I had not for a moment anticipated the kind of help I would need from my new nursing colleagues. It took only my first evening to recognize I had migrated to a foreign country. The west of Scotland is a land of Celtic mysticism, and those Celts and Picts and Hibernians treasure the unique nature of their ancient language. The first night I was assigned to my Neonatology rotation, I got an urgent phone call from Labour and Delivery.

"Can yeh gie heer reet quick, dooctar? This wee lassie joost had twin bairns. Nae more'n a poond each, I'm thunkin'. We havena' e'en weighed 'em. She stees wi' her gran and three other young 'uns in a Gorbals single-end."

I roused myself out of deep slumber, struggling to grasp the exact message behind her words—especially the mystifying information about where the patient was *steeing*. Surely this "wee lassie" was right there with the nurse—wasn't she? It wasn't till much later, as I grew comfier with my new surroundings, that I plucked up courage to ask a friendly nurse why she needed to know how many people shared how many rooms. The Gorbals of the seventies, she told me, was deemed the worst slum in Glasgow, perhaps in Europe. And a "single-end" meant a single tenement room with one outside privy shared with numerous other families. Self-evident, when I stopped to think about it, that these domestic details were vital to the way in which that nurse delivered her care.

Once I arrived in Accident & Emergency that night, it took me one long moment to figure out everything the nurse had told me on the phone. She was lifting brand new babies onto the scales; they weighed in at 980 and 950 grams respectively. As I pondered what on earth to do with these scarcely viable infants, I heard stirring behind me. I turned to see Mum curled up on a gurney, staring mutely at her newborns as though wondering where they had come from. I glanced at the chart at the end of the bed, searching for her first name.

"Annie, your boys are both very tiny. You know how far along you were?" She stayed mute. "Is your grandma around, I wonder?"

"She's doon in Casualty, dooctar, geein' the details," the nurse supplied. "She's to be hyin' back hoom to check on the young 'uns."

I caught the gist of her words and made my decision. "Annie, I'm going to phone our head doctor, ask her what she advises." I paused, arrested by the fearful eyes fixed upon me. "We'll keep your little ones comfy, don't you worry."

On the end of the phone, my boss promised to check on them "first thing—if they're still with us. Then we'll see what's to be done. The nurses can try syringing itty-bitty drinks into them, see if they can swallow."

I turned back to Mum, only to find she had fallen fast asleep. I glanced at my watch: ten to two. Still time to catch a couple of hours. Promptly at seven o'clock, the phone once more pulled me out of slumber.

"Heh theer, dooctar. Yeh wee twins are gooin' strong. Och, and we've moved them to their oon room in the Kiddies' ward. Mum being just a wee thing hersen, it seemed best. Thee're toughie wee bairns."

I felt profound relief to find my boss already at cribside. "Go ahead," she murmured to the babes' new nurse. I watched in astonishment as the nurse gently turned Babe 1's head to one side and sponged antiseptic over his temple, then wrapped a tourniquet around the infant's scalp that could fit an adult arm. A bluish tinge beneath the translucent skin signaled the presence of a vein. The nurse laid a 25-gauge needle—the smallest on offer—flat to the skin and dipped it downwards a fraction. There was a rapid flow of blood back into her syringe, and she withdrew a couple of milliliters of blood before deftly hooking up the intravenous line she had already prepared.

"Nice work, Rose," my boss told her. She turned to me. "The temple makes a good flat surface to rest your needle. And these neonatal nurses are your best resource if you're having a hard time getting an IV started."

I expected new trouble each morning, only to be greeted by the boys peacefully asleep on their sides, one at each end of their single crib. "Co-bedding" is the term commonly used in today's neonatal intensive care units. My mind flew back a quarter-century to sister Jane and me as tip-to-toe tinies sharing a bed on chilly winter nights. On day seven, I was startled to find Annie leaning over the crib side crooning softly. I tuned into the dulcet tones of the melody: maybe an old Scottish lullaby? I stood quietly as she addressed each of her babes in turn. Her Gorbals vernacular was impenetrable.

"Will tha luk a tha bairns' fuit . . . tha een." Then as each began to whimper: "Och, they're greetin'. . . . theer, theer, dinnah fash thissen."

I had not the faintest notion of what she was telling her boys, but it seemed too intimate a moment to disrupt her, let alone ask for translation. The nurse greeted me: "Reel champs, they are. We're reet prood of 'em."

"Why are mah bairns greetin'?" Mum quizzed her, clearly more comfy with one of her own.

"Och, they're maybe a wee chilled, hinnie. Don't goo upsittin' thissen."

The nurse's accent was almost as broad as Annie's, but I figured this was as good a time as any to learn a little of the Glaswegian vernacular, with this nurse right here to help.

"Um, I didn't quite catch what Mum was saying. I'd like to be able to, you know, understand her a bit better."

"Och, she talks the auld Glaswegian, dooctar. Let's see
. . . 'fuit' are 'feet' and 'een' would be 'eyes'. 'Greetin'—that's
'cryin'." What else? 'Dinna fash thissen' means 'don't upset yourselves.' Theer, ye'll be catchin' on in noo time."

I was rewarded with a broad grin from Annie. Uniting
across such a divide of language brought a lump to my throat.

A month after their birth, Annie was yet to name her two
boys. I was sitting beside her as she nursed twin 1 in her arms
and cautiously coaxed it with the small bottle of breast milk the
nurses had taught her to express. Our brief conversations com-
prised a lot of sign language, and I had come not to expect too
much more. Suddenly she addressed me.

"Wa's thee gien name?"

I looked blankly at the nurse.

"She means your Christian name, dooctar."

"Ah!" I grinned at both of them. "John."

"An' yer faither's?"

This time I caught on. "Richard."

"Och, thass it. John 'n Richard, I'm namin' 'em."

Such highly unlikely *sassenach* names for these dyed-in-
the-wool Scots-Irish boys—but I refrained from voicing my
thought.

"Annie, I'm honored you should choose our names.
Which is John and which is Richard?"

"I dunna. Yeh decide."

The lump was back in my throat.

CHAPTER 13

Conflict

In 1976, my deep respect for nurses bold enough to question a doctor's judgment was put to its strongest test. Dr. Jim Malpas, the head of medical oncology at Bart's, had invited me back to my alma mater, ten years after my graduation from its med school, to establish the first dedicated pediatric oncology department in Britain. The children were to be nursed on Kenton, the children's ward; and as a medical student I had had good reason to steer clear of Kenton. The reputation of its venerable nursing sister, who had been in total charge for several decades, had long caused any doctor below the rank of senior consultant to steer well clear. Sister Kenton was highly protective of her young charges and saw no reason to let trainee doctors, let alone the lowest of the low—us, the students—hone our fledgling skills at their expense.

So it was with some dismay, on returning to Bart's as a brand new consultant of thirty-four, that I found Sister Kenton still in total charge. Jim Malpas had tactfully informed me that his attempts to introduce even standard chemotherapy protocols for children with cancer had met with her stern resistance. He must have somehow come to the notion that his new hiree would be tough enough to weather the brunt of the inevitable storm. This was an image I was hard-pressed to picture. The tempest broke wide open early in my second week when I got a referral from an old colleague from my training years.

"Can you take a patient of mine? A four-year-old girl I admitted last night. She's got acute myeloblastic leukemia—has a white count of 100,000-plus. I'm thinking of that new protocol you developed in Glasgow. She'd be a great candidate."

At that time, acute myeloblastic leukemia—AML—was one of the last childhhood cancers to yield to the new chemo drugs, and the treatment we had developed in Glasgow, to which my friend was referring, was the most intensive ever tested. As I met with the little girl and her parents that afternoon, I was acutely aware of Sister Kenton hovering right at my left shoulder. Something in the sharp intakes of breath, the long pauses before she exhaled, told me I was in for a battle royal. And not just with this little one's leukemia.

"This treatment is certainly going to be very hard for Jennifer," I told Mum and Dad, "and for you too. I am very sorry to say that her leukemia is the kind that is hardest to treat. And the chemotherapy drugs we will need to give her are very strong. I want to assure you, though, that I've treated several children with this kind of leukemia, who have done very, very well. It's hard to believe, perhaps, but children are in many ways tougher than us grown-ups. Their young bodies handle the kinds of chemotherapy that you and I probably could not."

We were barely out of the room before Sister Kenton launched her attack. "Dr. Graham-Pole, you are giving these poor parents quite unjustified hope. No one has ever been cured of this form of leukemia. Certainly not the little ones it has been my sacred duty to nurse through their last moments. You are simply condemning her—and her parents—to unwarranted suffering. I have seen the terrible effects of the treatment you are proposing. I cannot prevent you from conducting these kinds of *experiments*"—she almost spat out the word—"but I wish to register my strongest objections to your proposed protocol."

The medical residents, the pediatric registrar, and two staff nurses had just shown up for rounds. They were very probably wondering if they should make themselves scarce until the storm passed. But I could sense their secret delight at witnessing this showdown between a venerable member of the nursing profession and an untempered newcomer to the Bart's consultant ranks overcame their inhibitions. They weren't going anywhere.

Meanwhile, I struggled to cool my rising irritation and find resort in reason. "Sister, my colleagues and I recently reported on fifteen children whom we treated for AML in Glasgow. I am glad to say that fourteen of them responded, and ten are alive up to five years later. You are absolutely right, this chemotherapy is of the most extreme, but anything less would simply postpone the inevitable."

At this moment, Jim Malpas appeared at the far end of the corridor. He had taken to joining us on rounds whenever he could get away, perhaps aware that I would welcome such reinforcements. As he drew level with our party Sister Kenton at once appealed to him.

"Dr. Malpas, I cannot believe what Dr. Graham-Pole is proposing for this poor little girl. I have registered my strongest objection to his proposal."

I already knew Jim for a skilled diplomat in tricky situations. "Sister, perhaps you might rustle up a cup of tea for John and myself in your office?"

We sipped for long moments in silence before Sister Kenton launched in. "Dr. Malpas, Dr. Graham-Pole has acquainted me with his plan of treatment for our new little patient—a patient who, I will add, has mere weeks, even days, to live. It is a treatment which I consider to be highly experimental and irregular—and quite beyond anything with which I and my nurses have familiarity. I am fully aware that the final decision rests with the doctors and the parents. I am also aware that it would be unethical of me to try to sway these poor young parents against your decision. If I must stand aside from a decision to which I fervently object, that I will do. But I would ask you to confer with Dr. Graham-Pole, and to bring your greater experience and, dare I say, wisdom to bear."

Jim paused for a long moment before answering, then carefully laid his teacup back down on its saucer. "Sister, I very much respect your feelings. And of course your own immeasurable experience and compassion." Another lengthy pause, then,

"However, I am personally responsible for hiring John. I did so because I knew he was breaking new ground in treating children with cancer of many kinds. I am particularly acquainted with the considerable success he has had with children with this form of leukemia using combination chemotherapy. It is, of course, far from without risk, but I believe he is fully justified in choosing this course. I know you will put your personal opinions aside and give every support to our medical staff."

I might not have been in the room. The two of them regarded each other in silence. Then Sister Kenton laid down her own teacup.

"Very well, Dr. Malpas. I shall say no more."

"Thank you, Sister. I know this isn't easy—for any of us. And thank you for a most refreshing cup of tea."

I followed Jim Malpas out, weak with relief. Would I ever develop such peacekeeping kills?

A month later, the little girl's temperature had finally fallen to normal, and she was sitting up in bed with her dolls propped on pillows on either side. Some God-given dispensation had allowed her to survive two rounds of my chemo protocol, while suffering a combination of relentless fever, burning mouth sores, and the temporary loss of her every blood cell. But all the signs were that her leukemia had responded completely.

At the end of my first year back at Bart's, Sister Kenton announced her intention to retire.

"I'm too old to change, Dr. Graham-Pole. These new treatments you are employing—well, I'll never accept them. They cause the children far too much pain and distress, and to what end? How many will ultimately survive?"

"I know we have had our differences, Sister. And you're absolutely right, the children do suffer a great deal—as do their families." I hesitated, wondering if we could perhaps find a little common ground. "But there are more and more treatments being developed, and we are getting many of the children back to living close to normal lives. At least for a time."

She shook her head. "Perhaps we must agree to differ, Dr. Graham-Pole."

At her retirement party Sister Kenton greeted me with more warmth than I had received from her that whole year.

"Dr. Graham-Pole, I'm happy to see you here. I thought perhaps, with our sporadic differences of opinion, you might decide to give my party a miss."

"I wouldn't have missed it for the world, Sister."

"I shall be retiring to my country home in Cornwall," she continued. "Perhaps you'll come and visit, bring me up to date with your latest experiments."

"I would be delighted to take you up on this kind invitation."

Very much a changing of the guard. While I had come to a resolute belief in the power of these new chemo drugs to do battle against the worst cancers afflicting children, I was only too aware how much suffering they caused. Sister Kenton was a remarkable and fearless advocate for what she believed to be right. And for her the *means*—these new and experimental chemotherapy protocols I had introduced—definitely did not justify the *end*.

CHAPTER 14

Stopping to Listen

I came early one morning to make rounds on a critically ill child with cancer who had been transferred to the pediatric intensive care unit. I listened as the head ICU physician scolded a new intern in a voice that could be heard throughout the ward:

"You've got to listen to the nurses! They know far more about your patients than you ever will. If you don't listen, every day and all day, you'll wrack up a bunch of avoidable deaths and disasters."

I had never heard it put so succinctly. Making me wonder just how many doctors, whether senior or junior, recognize the truth behind this senior physician's words. Nurses taught me almost everything important about my work—but only once I learned to stop and listen. It was my longtime nursing colleagues at Shands Children's Hospital, Nancy Dickson and Jan Luzins, who implanted in me that same chorus that I started to chant to every medical student and intern: "Listen to your *nurses*: they'll teach you everything!"

Tilda Shalof, a longtime ICU nurse and author of *A Nurse's Story*, tells the story of taking care of a scared and helpless intern faced with a critically ill patient in the early hours of one morning. He presented the picture of desperation as he stood at the foot of the bed, unable to raise his eyes to face her. Finally, he swallowed what remaining pride was left in him and broke the appalling tension.

"Help me. What should I do?"

"Transfer him to the cardiac unit. Now!"

Which was all it took.

McGill nursing professor Laurie Gottlieb calls nurses the *unsung* teachers of new doctors. They *catch* the early signs a patient is deteriorating, *correct* the interns' mistaken analyses of the signs and symptoms, and *cue* them how best they can intervene to put things right. All this in ways that rarely kill off the intern's last vestiges of self-esteem. More often, they help restore the self-confidence so vital to their being the best doctor they can be. Dr. Gottlieb has eloquently highlighted the devastating effects of doctors devaluing and undermining nurses and nursing.

Emergency rooms and intensive care units scared me from my first day of internship. Both departments were always choc-a-block with desperately ill patients needing highly competent and immediate care. It didn't take me long to swallow my pride and start asking the most approachable nurses for help, let alone how all the complex equipment worked. Are these brilliant, highly trained, and experienced frontline nurses ever acclaimed for all they have to offer? Only by the best doctors in the best hospital units—the ones who know from early on how well senior nurses supplement their book knowledge and technical skills with wisdom and insights. And how the resulting mutual respect between doctors and nurses can translate into the best possible patient care and outcomes.

Here are just a few lessons my nursing colleagues have taught me:

A good nurse is a mom and a coach and a nag;

Who else is there to clean up a helpless patient's sputum, blood, vomit, and feces?

Get to know something about your patient beyond their illness;

Listening and paying attention are treatments in themselves;

Use your hands and your brain and your heart in equal part;

Mortal illness teaches us compassion, faith, hope, gratitude, and humility;

Never stand silent in the face of unnecessary suffering;

To the questions your patient really wants to ask there are often no straight answers;

When giving good news, be happy; when shedding bad, be gentle;

Use the simplest and truest words to impart difficult or painful information;

Stress comes with the job: it can overwhelm, or it can exhilarate;

Your work can be distressing and depressing, and inspirational too;

Share your failures, your weariness, and your grief with a good listener;

Only if you remain calm and centred will you be of real help;

There is no limit to a patient's need, but there is to what you can give to them;

Even if your patient's outcome is good, they will always suffer along the way;

You may withdraw life-saving treatment, but never your loving care;

Talk to your patient like the most alive person you ever met, even when they're in deep coma;

Doctors make diagnoses and issue orders, but it's the nurses who really run things;

Efficiency with empathy—always;

There is always room for hope;

We're all potential patients; pray there's a good nurse there when it happens.

We doctors worry that constant closeness to illness and suffering, and allowing our feelings to show too openly, will impair our work. I think the truth is the opposite. Our presence and attention and touch and loving words can not only ease a patient's suffering as much as a shot of morphine; it can deepen our own emotional resilience and cognitive skills. It is healing medicine for both the one in the bed and the one sitting beside it.

Whatever course of action the doctor decrees—that whirlwind of too-often illegible orders—it is the nurse who carries it out. Nurses have their patients' lives right under their hands at all times. Even though much that they do to their patients is unpleasant—the repeated IV sticks, the never-ending round of pills, capsules, liquids, elixirs, suppositories, infusions of often noxious drugs, tubes to stick into every reluctant orifice, changing painful dressings—they strive to do it with efficiency and with empathy. It is the nurses who make people better.

CHAPTER 15

Ed and Alice

Soon after I arrived at Shands Hospital I became the pediatric director of our bone marrow transplant unit. And shortly met Ed. When he was a fourth-year student in psychology at the university Ed had developed a severe form of non-Hodgkin's lymphoma. It responded well to chemotherapy, and he remained in remission until he was twenty-five and in the third year of his graduate studies in health psychology. When his cancer recurred in several sites, my colleagues and I knew that his best, probably his only, chance for cure was a stem cell transplant. I met with Ed to talk about it.

"There's this wrinkle," he told me at once. "I'm planning on getting married—this coming weekend, actually."

"Well, you kept that close to your chest. So can you maybe rearrange your schedule?"

"Alice and I have talked about that. But then we started figuring out the odds against my coming out of your unit alive. Alice has all the data since you opened the unit. So no, we're not postponing."

Given the weight of therapy Ed had already had to bear, there was a very real possibility he wouldn't make it through our planned stem cell transplant. This highly aggressive treatment carried a significant risk of permanent damage to his liver, lungs, kidneys, psyche—you name it. I was about to embark on this tough pro-and-con conversation—should we go ahead or not?—when a penny clanged heavily to the floor: I knew only one Alice—and she was the stem cell unit's head nurse.

"Ed, do you mean the Alice I think you mean?"

Ed grinned broadly as he nodded. "I guess she kept it pretty quiet, too. But she's already made arrangements for Celia to take over." I knew only one Celia, too—Alice's immediate deputy on the unit. "Alice will be staying with me in my isolation room."

I reflected on all the implications of this unique situation. My first thought was that I had better be ready for one tough informed consent session. Alice was as well versed in the hazards of stem cell transplants as any of us doctors—and she wasn't one to hold back on voicing her opinions. Barely a week after their wedding I sat down with the newlyweds in our social worker's office for the formal consent process. They listened intently as I read through my five-page document that by mandate listed every aspect of the procedure. It was an ethical requirement to include every possible side effect—put more plainly, every single thing that could possibly go wrong. As I wound up and looked up at them both, Alice jumped straight in.

"John, what do you yourself think of Ed's chances? I mean, how big is the risk he'll get an infection he can't beat? And what about long term damage? Like, what are the chances we can still get pregnant?"

Ready for such pointed questions, I had armed myself with the latest research articles on stem cell transplant for this kind of cancer: a relapsed and heavily pretreated non-Hodgkin's lymphoma. But before I could muster my response, Alice swept on. It was like her first questions were almost rhetorical, and she didn't really want to hear my answers.

"I know all about the nursing coverage at night. But what about the medical staff? You don't have any transplant docs sleeping on the unit, right?"

"You're absolutely right, Alice. But the on-call attending is just a phone call away. Twenty-four-seven."

"You've got dedicated resident coverage through the night?"

"Well… pretty close." I was beginning to hedge. "There's a senior resident covering the oncology floor, with very ready access to the unit. And the ICU guys are only three floors above."

Then it was Ed's turn. "How about privacy? How much can Alice and I expect? We wouldn't be crazy about docs and nurses roaming in and out at all hours without so much as a by-your-leave."

Now we were way outside my purview. I wasn't about to quiz the two of them about exactly what conjugal rights they planned to exercise during Ed's prolonged spell of zero white cells and zero platelets. Sex in such a setting would be flirting with disaster, but I couldn't quite bring myself to ban such activity in these two honeymooners.

"Er... well... you'll of course have expert nursing care 24/7, but... "

Alice again: "John, the moment Ed and I step into that unit, I'll be *family* only, and absolutely not Ed's *nurse*. And I'll be doing my level best not to get in any nurse's way. But you know, too, that I'll be super-alert to anything I think needs immediate attention."

We chatted back and forth for thirty more long minutes, as I strived to keep my cool and not duck every and any challenge they threw at me. At last Ed sat back, slipped his arm tightly around Alice's shoulders, and eyed me full on.

"Thanks, doc. You haven't pulled any punches, but you sound pretty hopeful. Gives me the confidence I've been needing." He glanced at his new bride. "We're ready to sign."

The day they entered the unit, Ed gave Celia, as our new head nurse, copies of his power of attorney and personal directive. Both documents named Alice. They had also typed up their personal privacy requests.

"Look, I know your nurses have to check on me at least once a shift," Ed said to Celia. "Which of course is totally fine. And if they decide there's a problem, then I'm cool with whatever they need to do. But Alice will be with me twenty-four-seven—and she's seen me through plenty already. She's going to know right off if I'm in any kind of trouble."

I checked in on them before heading out for the night. I tried to picture my own wife going through this same life-threatening treatment, with me at her side every minute of every day and night for a month or more. Hardly the ideal way to start out your wedded life. But I hadn't the slightest doubt these two were heading into this whole thing with their eyes wide open. And if any young couple could come through this ordeal, it was Ed and Alice.

Four weeks later, they left their isolation room hand-in-hand to cheers from the staff. Within three months Alice felt it safe to leave Ed to complete his convalescence while she returned triumphantly to her role as nurse manager on the unit. Ed completed his graduate studies, defended his dissertation, and shortly afterwards joined the faculty of a distinguished university psychology department.

CHAPTER 16

Sharing Ourselves

It was nurses who taught me it was okay, even desirable, to share something of myself with my patients. I was desperately homesick when I arrived from London in Cleveland, Ohio, in 1978—and I found solace from an unanticipated source: my patients on the Rainbow Babies and Children's Hospital oncology ward. Those young ones had no notion that, totally unfamiliar as I was with American medicine, I was at sea without a sail. It was a big whoopee for them to test their best limey lines on me for my approval. The nurses caught onto my habit of sneaking back to sit on the children's beds at day's end while their parents grabbed the chance for a smoke. As I learned new games and watched silly TV shows, I shared with these young ones something of my life in England and my own childhood years. They didn't seem to notice the tears pricking at my eyelids.

Later on, I heard a young oncology nurse tell a teenager with advanced cancer how she had been there herself a few years earlier. Indeed she had; I was one of her doctors when she'd been on the receiving end of chemo at fourteen years old for the very same cancer. But my best memory of such sharing happened early on at Rainbow between a young nurse I will call Shanice and a black teenager, Dylan, who suffered from sickle cell disease. I was almost unacquainted with this horrid illness, so unprepared for how much pain and misery it could cause. Dylan had been hospitalized several days earlier in a sickle cell crisis and was drugged up with morphine for his brutal bellyache and bone pains.

He had maintained a stoical silence with me until Shanice showed up to check on him. She was a gorgeous black woman, with skin the colour of dark roasted coffee. Dylan lost all possible interest in me; his eyes became riveted on his new visitor.

"How's the pain, Dylan?" Shanice quizzed him. "Don't mind if I call you Dylan?"

He looked astonished, like no one had ever asked his permission about anything.

"Sure," he mumbled. "Well, I guess it's easing up some."

He hadn't been about to acknowledge this to me: male pride was plainly kicking in. Shanice moved to check his IV settings, then perched on the edge of his bed to take his vital signs.

"Is there anything I can do for you, Dylan? I haven't been around too many people with sickle cell, so maybe you can teach me some."

Now, why couldn't I have come right out and said that? Dylan's surly look had utterly vanished, replaced by an almost childlike softness. The young nurse's kindness had clearly got to him—that and her stunning looks. I eased back in my chair and let their conversation unfold.

"Yeah, sure. I know about everything there is to know. It's a killer, I can tell you that."

"D'you get many visitors, Dylan?"

"What's it look like? My mom, she's probably out with her latest. And Dad, he's been gone forever. And I can't hardly keep in touch with my buds, what with being in and out of this place."

"What about your girlfriend?"

His voice fell to a whisper. "I never had a date, No girl's ever going to want to go out with me."

"Don't you be so sure, Dylan. Lots of girls want to hang out with guys who've had more than their share of tough breaks."

He was close to tears. "Life sucks, you know?" he muttered.

Shanice stayed quiet, then reached out her hand and laid it on his arm. "I'm real sorry this all happened to you, Dylan. I hear you're in here quite a bit. I expect I'll be looking after you again."

"That'd be good."

"You know, there's something I don't usually share with my patients," she went on. "My last year in high school, I got this bad gut problem. Ulcerative colitis, they call it. Make a long story short, I had to have this massive surgery. And I ended up with a stoma. Around my nineteenth birthday, it was. Some birthday present, right?"

She promptly stood and pulled up her smock, then eased down the rim of her pants. A long pink scar snaked across her upper abdomen, and a colostomy pouch lay snug against her right side.

"That's my stoma—where the poop goes. The surgeons planned to hook me back up again, but it turned out it'd be too dodgy. So I'm stuck with it—like forever." She tugged her pants back up, dropped her smock in place, and grinned at us both. "But what I want to tell you, Dylan, it hasn't screwed up my social life one bit. One guy got turned off when he found out, but that relationship wasn't going anywhere anyway."

Dylan's face had lit up with a grin from ear to ear.

"Guess you never know what life's going to hand you," Shanice went on. "Just have to deal with it. And I know you can do that, Dylan. I'm rooting for you."

I was smiling to myself through the rest of my morning rounds. I had just been witness to a scene of healing in the form of loving words and a pretty face.

CHAPTER 17

Curing versus Healing

In my paper-publishing heyday, I was churning out articles as fast as I could submit them to the most prestigious journals out there. *Indexus Medicus*, the essential reference for aspiring medical academics, became my bible. Within its pages I would find reference to "the best journals in all relevant subject fields," per their promotional blurb. As a pediatric oncologist heavily involved in national clinical trials, I was starting to see my patients as dots on a survival curve.

When I exulted with a nurse friend about these improving figures, she quickly challenged me.

"Higher *cure* rates, you mean?"

"Right!"

"But what about all those late effects you hear about?"

I knew at once what she meant. We were recognizing that those very young children with leukemia we had routinely treated with cranial radiation, to stop the leukemia spreading to their brains, were growing up far shorter than their peers. And a blind twelve-year-old girl I was treating for osteosarcoma had already received intensive treatment in infancy for retinoblastoma affecting both her eyes. I had found references in *Indexus Medicus* to this same second cancer affecting several other such children.

"So are all these children really *healed*?" the nurse pressed me. "I mean, it's great that your chemo has cured them of their cancer, but at what cost? Can you really call them healed?"

Her words stayed in my mind as I finished up my day's work. Especially that last word—*healed*. She had pushed a button in me: how much credit could I claim for helping shift these survival curves upwards? I hurried to the medical school library to search for the word—and drew a total blank. There was no entry for *healing* in the entire *Indexus Medicus*. Another word came to mind that I had heard two nurses use: *holism*. Definitely not a word I had ever heard in med school; it just wasn't part of the curriculum. I didn't have to look to know *Indexus Medicus* would have no entry for it, but those nurses had been talking with animation about the idea. Something to do with the whole being greater than the sum of the parts. My nurse friend had taught me a hard but vital lesson: the only way to treat my patients was as complete and unique human beings; never, never, never as dots on a survival curve.

Judy became a favorite of mine on Shand's pediatric wards. Whenever I came to make rounds, she was often a welcoming face at the nurses' station, and never failed to fold me in a lingering hug. She had worked Peds her whole life and she would wrap her arms about me just like I was one of her charges. And she served another essential purpose for me: she knew more about my patients and their families than I ever would; and without breaking confidence she would share things she felt it would help me to know.

Her loving embrace was like a murmur of maternal lullaby, a kiss to make things better. Judy was a natural listener—a loving witness with ears attentive for any wounds of mind and spirit I might be suffering that morning. *Curing* wasn't a word you heard cross her lips. Instead, she taught me the larger meaning of *healing*—that of listening, witness, attention, and loving intent.

The word has its origin in wounds—physical, psychological, spiritual—often all three woven in one. The symbolism of the starched, pristine, maidenly uniform and cap may have disappeared, the bandage scissors replaced by scrubs and a stethoscope dangling doctor-like around the nurse's neck. But The Lady of the Lamp had it right, nursing remains an art form—the creative use of knowledge and skill for human betterment. In my early years as a med student and resident doctor, visiting hours were strictly limited—to twice a week for an hour.

So the nurses of those days became surrogate mothers—and often enough they mothered me too. As they greeted the year's wet-behind-the-ears interns each July, it was the floor nurses who helped these fledglings sort out the attending medical staff—by name, by rank, by reputation, and—most important—on a like-ability/approachability scale.

It's no accident that the French word for wound is *bless-ure*. We are all blessed, like it or not, with wounds—to our bodies, our minds, our spirits. I came to realize that that word, *healing*, is an intransitive verb: when wounded, we do our own healing— or strive to. It's not for others to heal us. Benjamin Franklin said, "God does the healing and the doctor takes the fee." Meanwhile, the nurses' loving care taught me the crucial role of a witness who lingered at bedside whenever the moment required it. That if the patient needed me to sit with them a while longer, this was always more vital than the demands of busy residents impatient to finish up on the wards so they could make it down to Radiology rounds by twelve sharp.

We doctors mostly place more value on skill than on empathy. Nurses taught me to always seek out the right balance between the two. That I needed to be sure my patients understood everything I told them about their illness and about its treatment.

"Now, are you sure you follow all I've told you? Is there anything else you want to know? There are no wrong or stupid questions, okay?"

Meanwhile, the nurses were performing those rote tasks that few doctors ever learn: drawing up meds, injecting, inserting, catheterizing, adjusting countless tubes. It was a rare day I had to deal with a patient's vomit, pee, or poop. We write our daily orders for chemo or boluses of morphine, but it is the nurses who push them into their patient's circulation, and are right on hand to deal with the inevitable side effects. I have ordered many thousands of doses of chemo, but rarely have I given thought to the training the nurses undergo to actually administer them: an IV push for some, a 24-hour infusion for others, adjusted to precisely the right rate of flow. While always remaining gowned and gloved to avoid the extreme toxicity of those chemo drugs. I prided myself as a young doctor on learning the art of locating almost invisible veins and establishing a stable IV line. But once that task was largely handed over to the nurses, I knew I could never match the skills of a nurse from Neonatology or a pediatric ICU unit. And how about interpreting the scribble of the doctor's orders, often enough not well thought through?

An experienced nurse can judge the severity of her patient's pain better than any numerical pain scale, just by spending a short time at bedside. Constant compassion is hard, often earns no thanks and often enough abuse from helpless, desperate, angry, hurting patients. Most of these patients are simply lonely and scared, need a loving hand to hold to lift them out of their abyss. That connection isn't so much friendship as a willingness to accompany them on their harrowing journey. And it is almost always the nurse—perhaps a very junior one—who is first at the bedside, and so the first responder, when a patient suffers a cardiac arrest and their heart stops dead. That nurse has to know instantly if the patient has a DNR status recorded in their chart; if not, she is the one who must call the code. Then she must start CPR singlehandedly while struggling simultaneously to calm the terrified family. Hard to imagine a lonelier place.

It was from nurses—all women in my early days—that I learned respect for the bodies of my patients, most especially the modesty of the many adolescent girls and young women I cared for. I needed to be sure they trusted me, that they knew I was totally *safe* as a young male doctor in charge of their care. Nursing is an essential mix of science and art—and you might well say the science is the easy part, that it's the art that is the most challenging. Nurses taught me to be open to my patient's emotional and spiritual pain without judging them and without depleting my own emotional energy. To talk in easy understandable ways, not in the doctor-speak we too often hide behind and which can put such "safe" distance between us. Too much documenting, quantifying, evaluating, and generating data risks losing sight of the human being before us. I cannot imagine nurses holding back sympathy from their patients to avoid their own emotional pain.

Yet nurses learn from their earliest teachings the science of observation and action—evaluating minute-to-minute changes in pulse rate and rhythm on a heart monitor. Most of what I have read about the work of nurses is the emotional support they offer to their patients. Too little is written about their scientific training and technical competence. Can I analyze a perilous degree of hypoxia from a patient's arterial blood gases, and know how to correct it with a touch of a knob? All the while moving to clean up the pee and poop spilt on the sheets? Half a nurse's work is wiping up the messes that bodies young and old, but too often helpless, generate. Nurses need the kind of physical stamina that was rarely asked of me as an intern, let alone as a professor. All I had to do was stay awake. I got to learn about new cancer drugs and draw up sexy new protocols, while it was the nurses who got to administer them and clean up the sometimes horrendous side effects.

What sticks most with me is how nurses taught me to sit and listen. I didn't have to be *doing* something every minute I was with my patient. "Stop and get to know them a little," is a mantra I heard many times—once I stopped to listen to my mentors. Yes, I took pride in my skills with a needle—but holding a wriggling three-year old for an LP without smothering him takes a greater skill.

Every patient in an intensive care unit is on some kind of life support. I never took an ICU-101 course on these machines, but nurses must study them up and down and inside out. How many orders have I written—typed or more often scribbled—that my nurse colleagues had to carry out, rarely raising a question? And who was there but the nurse to clean up the sputum, vomit, urine, feces from a helpless patient? If the stethoscope symbolizes the doctor, the bedpan symbolizes the nurse. Nurses work equally with their heads, their hearts, and their hands.

CHAPTER 18

Advocates for Bedside Art

What distinguishes art from science in healthcare? Our biomedical treatments are based largely on standard protocols: one size fits all. But artful medicine is never governed by protocol: it is tailored to fit each person we care for: the ideal setting for healing, the sorts of words we choose to use with them, how friendly or formal we are on first meeting, what music we might suggest for them, the best kind of pictures to hang on their walls. All these things vary vastly from patient to patient.

In 1990, when I had been working at Shands Hospital for almost ten years, I found myself wondering if professional artists could play a part in the care of my patients. And it was the nurses who at once embraced this—at that time—crazy notion. It started with Mary Rockwood Lane, a nurse-painter, who contacted me after I had published an article called "Art in Medicine" in *Housecalls*, a local medical magazine. When we first met in an off-campus bistro she recounted some painful life experiences of her own, and how making art had proved wonderful therapy for her.

"I think art can add a whole lot to medicine's focus on science and technology," Mary declared. "After all, children use art all the time to help deal with their traumas and catastrophes—painting and singing and dancing and so on. Why not grown-ups, too? Let's talk it up with the hospital nurses. We could have poets and musicians do performances in the hospital atrium, then move them on up to the wards. Bring them right to the patients' bedsides! Hey, why not?"

Which is how, in the spring of 1991, Mary and I came to create Arts in Medicine (AIM) at Shands. We chose the bone marrow transplant unit to bring our first artists to the bedside, partly because I was its co-director, but mostly because these patients were confined in semi-isolation for a month or longer. Helen Welsh, the unit's nurse manager, at once embraced the whole notion and flung open the doors to painters and poets and musicians and even dancers. She helped us launch this grassroots movement with no formal okay from the powers-that-be, and the unit nurses began to know their patients and families, and each other, on a totally new level. Helen and I developed a song-and-dance routine, which opened with Helen singing:

"I'm just the nursing Soop
And I jump through Doctor's hoop
And I clean up all the poop
Boopy-ti-boop, boopy-ti-boop, boopy-ti-boop. ... "

An unknown photographer captured a playful moment between Helen and me, which you can see on the back of this book.

It was always the nurses who advocated for art and artists to work at a particular patient's bedside. Through some kind of nursing underground, the word spread and other units began to embrace this new movement. Meanwhile my medical colleagues either ignored it entirely or at best paid lip service.

It was through AIM that I formed a special friendship with a male nurse, Steve Kavalin. Steve showed up one Friday afternoon with his camera at a music and poetry presentation in the hospital atrium. He was a nurse anesthetist—the first I had met. He began appearing at many AIM events to capture moving images at bedsides, in clinics, and in many places where our performances took place. He and I started hanging out together, playing endless games of racquetball, and making trips to Florida's east coast for wonderful soft-shell crab dinners, washed down with schooners of beer. Steve became a close friend at a time when I was separated from my wife and very much in need of such a buddy.

But however many men become nurses, and however many women enter the medical profession, for me the two professions will always retain their male and female archetypes.

Women are our natural healers—as nurses, midwives, and artists. Doctors and nurses have quite different tools: knives and drugs versus thermometers and dressings. Doctors lean against doorways, nurses sit on beds. The nurse's artform is her gift of time and of love—and this is an ancient art: Florence Nightingale saw nursing as requiring as much study, skill, and application as that of a sculptor or a painter. As my interest in the art of healing deepened, and I watched nurses welcoming artists to their hospital wards, I came to recognize nursing as an ancient and autonomous profession quite distinct from anything we physicians had to offer.

Nurses have been much quicker than us doctors to grasp the essential unity of mind, body, and spirit, and the subjective experience of illness over the objective description of disease. While physicians continue to work, mostly at a distance, with empirical scientific data, nursing practice concerns itself with immediate bedside experience. Nurses hear the stories their patients crave to tell them; this in turn helps these patients make sense of their situation, which cannot fail to promote their healing. Nurses strive to treat their patients always as people, never as machines—dodging that trap physicians all too often fall into. But nurses, too, are challenged today to integrate the art and science of their practice into our frenetic healthcare environments. They have little or no time to grieve the death of a patient they may have nursed for weeks or even months.

On two memorable occasions my nurse colleagues advocated directly for my own health. When I started work at Shands in 1981, Jan Luzins and Nancy Dickson were part of our pediatric oncology team, and I quickly learned to tune into their *grace notes*: brief, quiet suggestions to complement my decisions as the doctor in charge. I was brand new on the University of Florida faculty, and I knew these two nurses had much to teach me. I was making rounds with Jan one morning when I became aware of a sharp pain in my left eye. I had woken with it early that morning but had thrust it out of my mind.

"What's wrong, John? You didn't even open that chart."

She was indicating the patient notes on the trolley we were wheeling ahead of us, holding the charts that contained our patients' medical histories—their life stories. She was standing in front of me as though preventing further forward traffic, and I just couldn't look directly at her. The very daylight was suddenly too painful. I was aware of the gentle concern in my nurse-friend's voice and felt unaccustomed tears well up in my throat.

"Something's wrong with my eye. I don't know… it's so painful."

"Come and sit, let me take a look."

She took my hand and led me to two chairs in the nursing station, like I was her child and she was going to kiss my booboo better. I felt her cool hands on my face, a tender lifting of my left upper eyelid. I had to quickly shut it against the light as tears flooded forth.

"John, I'm going to call Bill, have him take over from you. We need to get you down to the eye clinic."

My tears were flowing freely, whether from the excruciating pain in my eye or Jan's tenderness. Within minutes she had led me to the elevator and walked me to the ophthalmology clinic on the first floor beyond the atrium. I could never have found the place on my own. She spoke quickly and quietly to the nurse who came out to greet us and whom Jan knew well.

"One of the docs is going to take a look in a few minutes, John. I'll just sit with you till things get taken care of."

Thank you, Jan. Thank you for knowing what to do. For taking over. For taking care of me.

Soon after I recovered from what proved to be *Acanthamoeba keratitis*, a rare parasitic infection that had invaded the cornea of my left eye, probably from lubricating fluid for my contact lenses, I had another occasion to bless a ministering nurse angel. Cathy, a motherly woman in her forties, was our regular nurse in the pediatric oncology clinic that I ran every Tuesday. She was in charge of checking the patients in and collecting their vital signs. The children loved her, but the littlest ones were often upset when it came to having their blood pressures checked. It was the tight pressure of the cuff on their upper arms that bothered them. So during the early morning rush I would perch on one of the smallest children's chairs and have Cathy read off my own BP.

The third time she checked it she took me aside. "John, have you seen a doctor about your blood pressure?"

"No. Why, is it up?"

"It is, and it was last week too. 150 over 105—I made a note of it because it bothered me. So I'm glad I got to check it again."

I blew her off. "It's just because I've got a specially heavy clinic today—dunno when I'll get out of here."

"Okay, well, I'm going to keep an eye on it. I want you to come by on Friday afternoon when your day is winding down. I'm making you my special project."

Sure enough, my blood pressure was still as high the next time Cathy checked it.

"You need to see your doctor, John." She eyed me quizzically. "You do have one, don't you?"

I looked sheepish.

"You don't, do you? You doctors," she chided me. "You think you're immortal! I don't know any nurses who don't get regular check-ups. There's a very good guy in the family practice department. You'll like him."

Two weeks later Cathy's recommended physician confirmed her diagnosis, ran an EKG and a bunch of blood tests, and started me on medication for my hypertension. I sometimes wonder if it would ever have been diagnosed until a heart attack or a stroke felled me in my seventies. I kept a weekly check on my blood pressure, and both Cathy and I were gratified to see it drop within a few weeks into a normal range.

Thank you, too, Cathy, for your wise and loving care.

CHAPTER 19

Marshmallows

The writer E.B.White accused our society of being suspicious of anything *non-serious*. Thank the stars, then, for humour. I had a teenage patient with advanced cancer tell me after I had given him some none too hopeful news: "Lighten up, doc, I don't need solemn doctors about me." A good lesson from a wise child.

One busy Friday, Betsy, the nurse manager on the PICU, beckoned me into her office as I was wrapping up rounds for the day. I knew tensions had been running high on her unit after a series of tragic outcomes. She and I had been buddies for years, and it crossed my mind she might want to get something off her chest.

"I've called a meeting of all my nursing staff," she said without preamble. "They'll be here in a few minutes. Can you stick around?"

"Why pick on me?"

"Well, you're up here a lot," Betsy responded. "And you're a good bit older, too."

"It's that obvious, is it?"

"Oh, you're still a kid to me. But they don't know that."

Betsy was referring to the seven nurses about to descend on her office. We both giggled—she might be in her late thirties, and I wouldn't see sixty again.

"Okay. I guess I've been around the block a few times. And I've probably got twenty years on most of the ICU docs, too."

"I haven't invited them, by the way. Just the nurses and you. They'll think you're here because of Sandra."

Sandra—the most recent child to die on the unit—had been a patient of mine. She had a glioblastoma—an almost universally fatal brain cancer. The little girl had lapsed into coma before she got transferred up from our pediatric cancer ward; she hadn't been feeling much of anything when they put out yet another code within an hour of her reaching the PICU. It turned out she had already taken her final breath.

"They don't have to know you're really here to hold my hand if the going gets rough," Betsy added. "We've lost five children in the past two weeks."

I knew what she was getting at. Betsy had called this meeting specifically because of tensions building between the nurses and the ICU docs—and some of these nurses could be hard to handle. Rose—the nurse caring for Sandra when she died—had come close to boiling point with the attending doc and his over-heroic efforts. Her opinion, anyway.

A brief knock on the door and the nurses filed in. They must have gathered together outside to reinforce their solidarity. I knew all seven by sight, most by name, and I sensed they all knew me. There were only two vacant chairs, one large enough for two, so the other four sat on the carpet and leant up against the legs of the ones in the chairs. There was some friendly jostling as the room filled to capacity. Things settled into an expectant silence, then Betsy looked around at everyone in turn.

"It's been real hard up here lately, we all know that. So this is just a time for y'all to vent, share your feelings, whatever you need to do."

Rose spoke up fast. "Too right it's been hard. Some of those kiddies were never going to make it, Betsy. But the docs just can't seem to get it sometimes."

Annie picked it up. "Yeah, with that last code—as soon as Dave finally called a halt, he just went straight back on rounds. Like nothing had happened. Left it to the poor little intern to break the news to Mum. Jeez, he's an unfeeling brute."

Annie's outburst gave everyone permission to blow the lid off.

"I never thought it could get this bad…"

"Five deaths in—what, a week and a half…"

"Some of those guys just don't know when to stop…"

"Maybe we should have called a few ethics consults…"

"My boyfriend's getting pissed at me, crying every night…"

"Mine took off. I'm about ready to quit…"

The cacophony persisted for several minutes. Two nurses began crying freely, feeling the unspoken permission to vent feelings too long held in check. A sense of release surfaced around the room, and Betsy let things run, knowing they needed to do this. As things quietened, she stretched out both hands to the two closest to her, and the rest took the cue, hugging and holding hands.

Then tears gave way to brief grins. I laid a hand on the shoulder of Mia, whose back was propped against my knees. She freed her own hand, raised it to grasp mine, returned my squeeze. My throat thickened. I grabbed a handy box of tissues and blew my nose, then offered the soggy mess to Mia. Grins became guffaws. These nurses knew well the crucial resource of laughter, even— or especially—in an intensive care setting. Betsy took time to embrace everyone with her beaming smile.

"Thanks for coming—all of you. And feeling you could say your pieces. We've all got a lot of crying to do. To hell with boyfriends who can't hack it. There really are some good men out there!" More giggles. "Hey, maybe those attending docs could use a few hugs. Can't hurt, might help!"

Rose looked at Betsy like she was about to blow off the very idea, but she stayed quiet. Maybe she was even picturing the scene?

"Just be sure you don't blame yourselves," Betsy went on. "Like things could have turned out okay if you'd just done things a bit differently. Second-guessing can keep you awake all night." She paused to take in everyone in turn. "Just know you did your best. I'm really happy you all decided to work here."

Which brought fresh sniffles around the room. None of the nurses had launched any more attacks on the ICU docs after their first few salvos. The anger had surfaced fast and hard, then quickly given way to free expressions of grief. As if everyone knew this was the core thing, this big knot of helplessness and heartache. That shedding it was what this precious time was for. Not for blaming absentee doctors for their decisions and actions.

Rose freed up a hand to tear open a couple of packs of marshmallows. They made the rounds along with someone's flask of Gatorade. People grabbed handfuls like they hadn't eaten in a week. Candy quickly started spilling. After a bunch of face-stuffing and chomping, one suddenly flew through the air and caught Rose in the chest. Someone yelled, "Marshmallow fight!" cuing Rose to hurl several back in the general direction the first missile had been launched. At once everyone was scrambling for larger handfuls and slinging them in random directions. Tears became guffaws of laughter.

After several minutes of bedlam, the energy started to stall. Rose finally yelled out, "Okay, eat 'em all up now!"

There were no takers—most of the marshmallows had gathered a coating of rug or got ground under knees or butts. The brief feast over, we set about working with damp cloths from the bathroom, wiping off bits of goo from chairs and carpet.

"Anyone need their butt wiped?" Annie offered.

As I left, I checked my watch. Less than an hour—not too long out of a 168-hour week. And nobody was going to burn out today. Someone's boyfriend might even get a big grin and a spicy kiss tonight.

CHAPTER 20

Pegasus

When we first opened *Pegasus*, our children's hospice and palliative care unit, I knew I could learn everything I needed from the nurses staffing the adult hospice. On my first visit my attention was caught by harp music filling a patient's room. It was coming from the CD player sitting on a small stool by the door.

"You've heard of music thanatology?" asked Christine, the nurse given the task of mentoring me about the particular ways of hospice care.

"Can't say I have."

"Well, we found out a while back that harp music and chanting can be very soothing. Some musicians get professional training, but recorded music works pretty well. I've made a couple of different playlists."

When the patient, Mr. Peters, grew agitated, as Christine told me happened with many people towards the end, she would play a specially soothing piece on the CD, and the lines of his face would relax before he fell into a slumber. One time, he opened his eyes to tell us sleepily, "Comfort food for the ears."

Christine taught me about massage oils. She handed me a small plastic bottle half-filled with oil. "This mix of lavender and peppermint is my favorite. Peppermint's an analgesic, you know, John. The ancients used it. Keeps me calm, too, inhaling the aroma."

She went on to teach me the gentle rhythm that worked best for massaging a wasted body. She would kneel down at the bedside in the ancient attitude of prayer to carry it out. She also taught me how best to roll a patient from side to side, change the sheets and pillowcases while barely disturbing them, and clean coated gums with lemon and glycerine swabs. Mr. Peters had taken a particular liking to frozen ginger popsicles, and his wife kept a regular supply in the freezer.

There came the time when he couldn't make it to the bathroom. I loved the matter-of-fact yet deeply compassionate way Christine eased the old guy into diapers. He had that far-off look of one very soon to leave us, but he was with it enough that Christine's suggestion bothered and even embarrassed him.

"We're all born into diapers, and most of us die in them," Christine told him gently. "And one of us will be here to switch them out whenever."

Which got a grin and a brief look—the way Mr. Peters might have eyed any young woman in his heyday. He even managed to joke about it: "It's not dying I mind, but if I'd known it meant diapers..." Both Christine and I knew we'd convinced him it would be a lot easier on all of us. He was eating and drinking less and less, so it was no big deal to change him. Over those first days of my orientation to the unit I watched Mr. Peters' breath grow fainter and more episodic, his skin colour fading to white, then to dullish blue. Until his heartbeat finally faded completely as he slipped into the warm womb of death. Christine leaned in to kiss his forehead.

"It's just his aura we're feeling now," she murmured to me.

She and I had shared life stories while the rest of the family slept. It was only much later that I took note of the time typed on the death certificate: 4:15 a.m. I had dozed off in my chair when Christine laid a gentle hand on my arm to tell me it could happen any moment.

"Many people die at night. Perhaps most. That's why I'm a night owl," she said. "It's almost as if they take their loved ones' sleeping as permission to enter their own eternal slumber."

When it became clear the end was nigh, Christine stayed a good part of each day and often well into the night. She would take short breaks to head home for an hour or two to check on her husband and her eight-year-old daughter.

"He hasn't had a thing to eat for days," I said to her once. "He's not even swallowing fluids. Surely he must be hungry for something—or at least thirsty."

"I don't think he's feeling much hunger or thirst at this point," she told me. "People used to think we should give IV fluids when patients stopped drinking. But it isn't necessary or even beneficial. The big thing is to keep his mouth clean and moist."

Christine was perfectly fitted for the role she had trained for. Aware and caring instantly for her patients' bodily needs; alert to how the family was coping; guiding, teaching, consoling, answering questions, lightening things up when the chance arose. Gently and so competently washing and robing the body after death. She was tireless and deeply loving: a spiritual presence.

In addition to the children's hospice, I began running the new palliative care program at Shands, and I had a nurse practitioner to make daily rounds with me. Early on, I had a referral from the Neonatal Intensive Care Unit to see a baby with anencephaly, a birth defect in which the major parts of the brain, scalp and skull don't form as the baby is developing in the womb. When I first saw baby Eddie, his dad Sam was more than ready to let him go. But Rose, Eddie's mom, wasn't there yet.

"No. No, not yet. I need a sign," she cried to me when I let her know it wouldn't be long. Sam looked set to press his case, but instead he closed his eyes as though in prayer. Then: "I understand, Rose. We'll wait on a sign."

The other family members also closed their eyes. Meanwhile, the ICU staff had no alternative, so they got ready to intubate the baby, still less than twenty-four hours old, and hook him up to a ventilator. Normally this is a routine enough procedure in the Neonatal ICU, but it took more brute force than skill to get the endotracheal tube in place and inflate Eddie's congested little lungs with enough oxygen to keep him alive. An hour later in the grocery store aisle I got an urgent page.

"The tube's out, John," the ICU nurse yelled down the phone, startling several of my fellow shoppers. "It's bedlam, we can't get Rose calmed down enough to decide if she wants us to keep on trying. Get here as soon as you can, will you?"

By the time I arrived back in Eddie's pod, everyone was embarked on the bloody business of getting another breathing tube down his tiny windpipe. Rose insisted on staying right beside his crib, which wasn't helping matters. But as soon as I entered the pod, she flung herself on me and moaned, "Stop! Stop! It's the sign!"

"Are you sure now, Rose? It looks like they just got the tube back in place again."

"I'm sure. It's the sign. You don't have to go on any-more."

We gathered in a semicircle as the ICU attending doctor prepared to draw out the fresh endotracheal tube—this time for good. Rose never wavered again in her decision and sat quietly waiting with Sam and their three other children. One of the nurses injected a massive dose of Fentanyl into Eddie's IV line to make sure he would be quite oblivious. As the senior doctor gradually drew the tube out from his trachea, Eddie gasped just once before his whole body darkened. I could still hear his heart-beat for a minute, maybe a little longer, before it finally stopped and never beat again.

Between them, Rose and Sam gathered Eddie up into Rose's arms, murmured to him and stroked his head as his sib-lings grouped themselves around her. Rose cried a few more tears, then looked around at us caregivers. All at once she broke into a big beam.

"Why don't y'all hold him?"

Taking her cue, we allowed ourselves a collective smile. I stepped up to lift Eddie from Rose, then passed him on to the nurse beside me So it continued for several minutes. Later, I reflected that in the end it had been a good death, that there had been some purpose to Eddie's short and tragic life. What I remember most is all the hugging, tears, laughter, then more rounds of hugs. I had never before nor since hugged so many fellow caregivers. For a short time, our intensive care unit was transformed into a sacred place of community. Of communion.

Once we started getting regular referrals to the pediatric hospice program, we rarely had to admit the children into the actual hospice unit. Instead, I made frequent house calls—something I hadn't done since making rounds as a teenager in Yorkshire with my uncle-doctor Ken. One morning my beeper buzzed as I was finishing my hospital rounds. It was Cendra, our new hospice nurse.

"I'm at Marie's house, John. The little one with the brain tumor. Her headache's getting steadily worse. I need a stat order to up her morphine."

This was a first: ordering IV narcotics to a nurse on the phone from fifty-odd miles away.

"What's she on?"

"2 mg every four—I want to go straight to 3."

"Agreed, and another milligram in ten minutes if she needs it."

Thirty minutes later another buzz. I was still in my car, hurrying towards the house keeping barely to the speed limit.

"She's still writhing. Can I up it some more?"

"Remind me—what weight is she?"

"Just over 15 kg."

The usual dose being 0.1mg/kg, we were already at over twice that. But Marie had been fading fast, and on my last visit her parents had been more than ready to let her go.

"Go with 4 mg, and another 2 every thirty. How are Mom and Dad doing?"

"They're ready. More than."

"And you?"

"I'm okay." I'd never heard Cendra show weakness, or even offer a complaint. She added, "The local pharmacy's only got one IV dose left. A van's coming from Shands with supplies."

"I'll be with you in twenty minutes. 5 mg every ten till then."

When I arrived, Mom was cradling Marie in her arms while Dad and Cendra held Mom between them. Marie had died five minutes before I got there. Cendra looked weary but calm.

"It was peaceful at the end, John."

I reflected that between us we had brought this little girl's life to a quite intentional end. But it was Cendra who had done all the heavy lifting.

Afterword

That beautiful word *grace* derives from the Latin *gratia*, and means bestowing a service, or performing a gracious act that merits thankfulness. In a religious sense, it originally meant divine virtue or approval, and also a celebration or song of praise to render thanks to the gods. The closely related word *gracious* implies one who offers courtesy, compassion, generosity of spirit, and mercy.

Through their every random act of kindness, nurses make infinite contributions—*grace notes*—to our gift economy. And this at a time when healthcare risks being enslaved to the corporate markets.

Thank you, everyone of you.

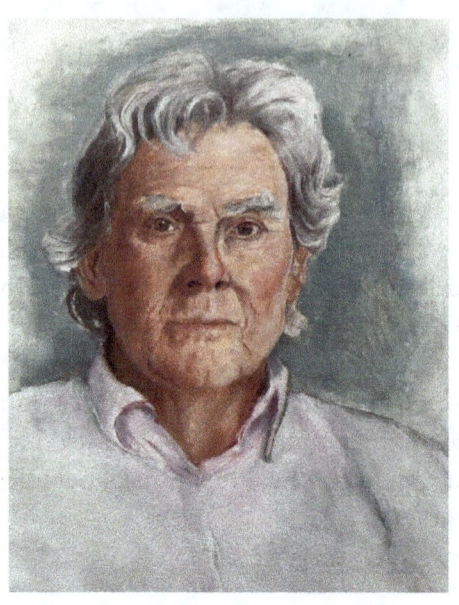

John Graham-Pole is a retired professor of pediatrics. He was a clinician, teacher, and pioneer researcher in the field of childhood cancer for forty years. Educated in Britain, he co-founded Shands Hospital Arts in Medicine (artsinmedicine. ufhealth.org) and the Centre for Arts in Medicine at the University of Florida (https://arts.ufl.edu/academics/center-for-arts-in-medicine/), now among the world's leading arts-and-health organizations. The university has named both a lectureship series in pediatric palliative care and a student scholarship in arts-medicine in his name.

He is the author of twelve works of fiction, non-fiction, and poetry. His most recent publications are *Songlines*, the third in a trilogy of novels inspired by young people with cancer, *Healing by Intent*, his second medical memoir, and *Illness and The Art of Creative Self-Expression*, an extensively updated reissue of his 2000 work on creativity as an essential element for our health.

He lives in Nova Scotia with his wife, Dorothy Lander, where in 2018 they co-founded HARP: The People's Press (www.harppublishing.ca), a multimedia publishing house dedicated to exploring how the arts can enhance our individual and communal health. His personal website is www.johngrahampole.com and he can be found on Facebook and Linked-In.

www.ingramcontent.com/pod-product-compliance
Lightning Source LLC
Chambersburg PA
CBHW071018120626
46546CB00003B/1140